MW00607795

It's easy to get lost in the cancer world

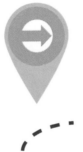

Let NCCN Guidelines for Patients® be your guide

✓ Step-by-step guides to the cancer care options likely to have the best results

✓ Based on treatment guidelines used by health care providers worldwide

✓ Designed to help you discuss cancer treatment with your doctors

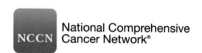

NCCN Guidelines for Patients® are developed by the National Comprehensive Cancer Network® (NCCN®)

NCCN

✓ An alliance of leading cancer centers across the United States devoted to patient care, research, and education

Cancer centers that are part of NCCN:
NCCN.org/cancercenters

NCCN Clinical Practice Guidelines in Oncology (NCCN Guidelines®)

✓ Developed by doctors from NCCN cancer centers using the latest research and years of experience

✓ For providers of cancer care all over the world

✓ Expert recommendations for cancer screening, diagnosis, and treatment

Free online at
NCCN.org/guidelines

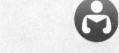

NCCN Guidelines for Patients

✓ Present information from the NCCN Guidelines in an easy-to-learn format

✓ For people with cancer and those who support them

✓ Explain the cancer care options likely to have the best results

Free online at
NCCN.org/patientguidelines

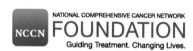

and supported by funding from NCCN Foundation®

These NCCN Guidelines for Patients are based on the NCCN Guidelines® for Primary Cutaneous Lymphomas (Version 1.2021, October 12, 2020).

NCCN Foundation seeks to support the millions of patients and their families affected by a cancer diagnosis by funding and distributing NCCN Guidelines for Patients. NCCN Foundation is also committed to advancing cancer treatment by funding the nation's promising doctors at the center of innovation in cancer research. For more details and the full library of patient and caregiver resources, visit NCCN.org/patients.

National Comprehensive Cancer Network (NCCN) and NCCN Foundation, 3025 Chemical Road, Suite 100, Plymouth Meeting, PA 19462 215.690.0300

Endorsed by

The Leukemia & Lymphoma Society
The Leukemia & Lymphoma Society (LLS) is dedicated to developing better outcomes for blood cancer patients and their families through research, education, support and advocacy and is happy to have this comprehensive resource available to patients. lls.org/patientsupport

To make a gift or learn more, please visit NCCNFoundation.org/donate or e-mail PatientGuidelines@nccn.org.

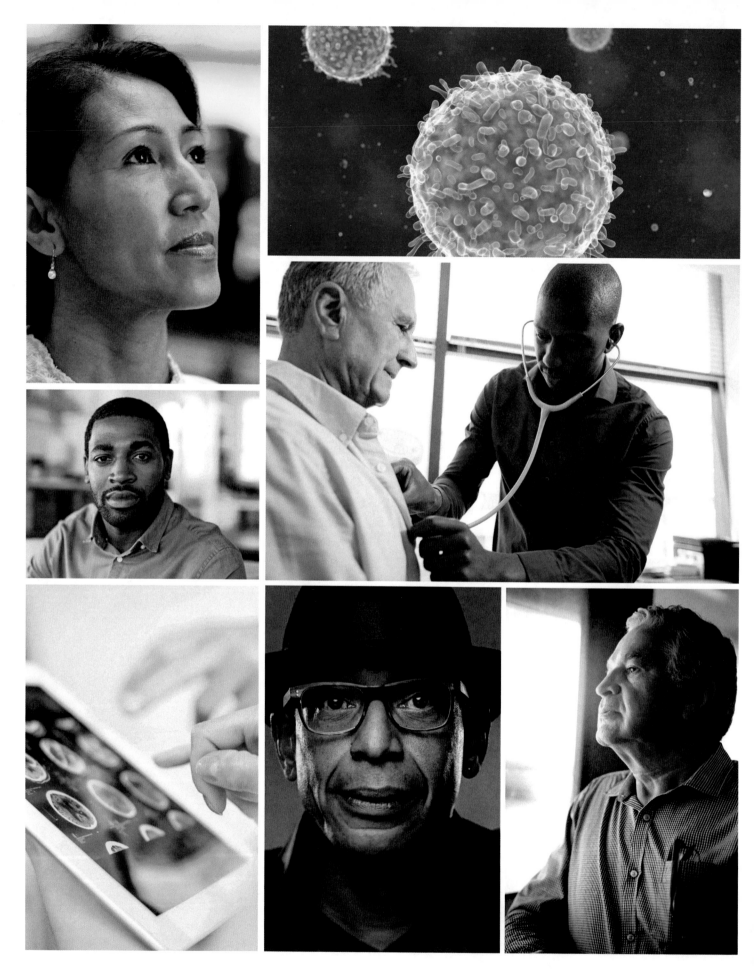

Contents

6   PCL basics

12   Testing for PCL

25   Treating PCL

33   PCBCL

41   PCLPD

45   Cutaneous ALCL

51   LyP

56   Making treatment decisions

69   Words to know

71   NCCN Contributors

72   NCCN Cancer Centers

74   Index

1
PCL basics

7   The lymphatic system

8   Lymphocytes

9   Primary cutaneous lymphomas

11   Review

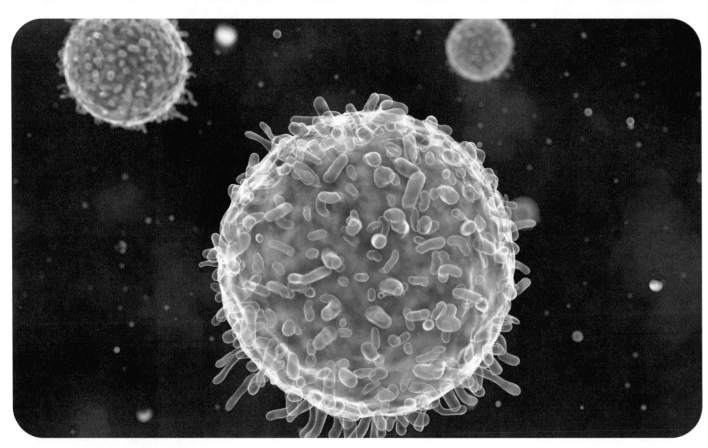

Primary cutaneous lymphomas (PCLs) are a group of B-cell and T-cell non-Hodgkin lymphomas. Non-Hodgkin lymphoma is a cancer of a type of white blood cell called a lymphocyte. In PCL, abnormal lymphocytes cause skin lesions. Although the skin is involved, the skin cells themselves are not cancerous.

The lymphatic system

Lymphoma is the most common type of blood cancer. It affects the lymphatic system. The lymphatic or lymph system is a major part of the body's immune system. It is a germ-fighting network of tissues and organs that includes the bone marrow, spleen, thymus, lymph nodes, and lymphatic vessels.

Lymphatic vessels are a network of thin tubes that carry lymphatic fluid (lymph) and white blood cells into all the tissues of the body. Lymph gives cells water and food. White blood cells help fight infection and disease.

As lymph travels throughout your body, it passes through hundreds of small bean-shaped structures called lymph nodes. Lymph nodes make immune cells that help the body fight infection. They also filter the lymph fluid and remove foreign material such as bacteria and cancer cells.

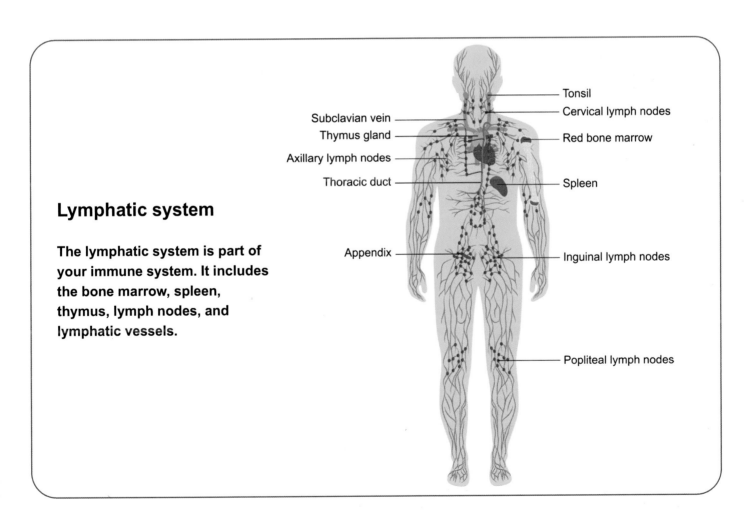

Lymphatic system

The lymphatic system is part of your immune system. It includes the bone marrow, spleen, thymus, lymph nodes, and lymphatic vessels.

Subclavian vein
Thymus gland
Axillary lymph nodes
Thoracic duct
Appendix

Tonsil
Cervical lymph nodes
Red bone marrow
Spleen
Inguinal lymph nodes
Popliteal lymph nodes

Lymphocytes

A lymphocyte is a type of white blood cell. White blood cells fight infections. Lymphocytes are found in both blood and lymph tissue. Lymph tissue includes lymph vessels and lymph nodes.

There are 3 main types of lymphocytes:

> ➤ B lymphocytes or B cells make antibodies. An antibody is a protein.

> ➤ T lymphocytes or T cells help kill tumor cells and help control immune responses.

> ➤ Natural killer (NK) cells have granules (small particles) with enzymes that can kill tumor cells or cells infected with a virus.

Primary cutaneous lymphomas can be a result of abnormal B cells, T cells, or NK cells. Lymphocytes normally grow in response to infection or inflammation. When they grow on their own, they can develop into a lymphoma.

B cell

B cells produce antibodies that are used to attack invading bacteria, viruses, and toxins. The antibody molecules latch onto and destroy invading viruses or bacteria.

T cell

T cells are direct fighters of foreign invaders and also produce cytokines, which help activate other parts of the immune system. The T cells destroy the body's own cells that have been taken over by viruses or that have become cancerous.

NK cells

NK cells recognize and kill virus-infected cells, detect and control early signs of cancer, and protect against disease. NK cells can "remember" certain virus cells for many years and fight to keep the body from being infected again.

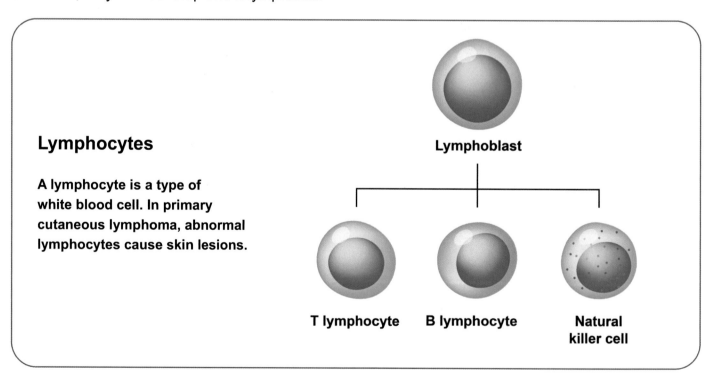

Lymphocytes

A lymphocyte is a type of white blood cell. In primary cutaneous lymphoma, abnormal lymphocytes cause skin lesions.

Lymphoblast

T lymphocyte   **B lymphocyte**   **Natural killer cell**

Non-Hodgkin lymphoma

Lymphoma starts in lymphocytes. Non-Hodgkin lymphoma (NHL) can be formed from either B-cell, T-cell, or NK-cell lymphocytes. Primary cutaneous lymphomas are a type of NHL.

For more information on lymphomas, see NCCN.org/patientguidelines.

Primary cutaneous lymphomas

Primary cutaneous lymphomas (PCL) or skin lymphomas are a rare group of NHLs that develop in the skin. At the time of diagnosis, PCL is not found in any other areas of the body. Skin lymphoma is not a type of skin cancer. Skin cancer develops from skin cells. PCL develops from abnormal lymphocytes.

PCL is a chronic, but treatable condition. PCL causes skin lesions that are often itchy and scaly. Lesions may appear red, purple, or brown, and can be lighter in color than the surrounding skin. It might show up as more than one type of lesion and on different parts of the skin (often in areas not exposed to the sun). Some skin lymphomas appear as a rash.

> A lymphocyte is a type of white blood cell. In primary cutaneous lymphoma (PCL), abnormal lymphocytes cause skin lesions.

Cutaneous B-cell lymphomas

Cutaneous B-cell lymphoma (CBCL) appears as a nodule under the skin that might look like small pimples called papules. CBCL is not a systemic (widespread internal) disease.

Types include:

> - Primary cutaneous marginal zone lymphoma (PCMZL)
>
> - Primary cutaneous follicle center lymphoma (PCFCL)
>
> - Primary cutaneous diffuse large B-cell lymphoma, leg type (PC-DLBCL, leg type)

Most primary cutaneous B-cell lymphomas (PCBCLs) are indolent or slow-growing.

Cutaneous T-cell lymphomas

Cutaneous T-cell lymphoma (CTCL) is a rare form of cancer that develops when T lymphocytes, which are white blood cells that fight infection, grow and multiply uncontrollably in the skin. This chronic condition requires ongoing care and management. CTCLs are treatable and sometimes curable.

CTCL can cause rash-like redness, slightly raised or scaly round patches, plaques, and sometimes skin tumors. Most CTCLs are indolent (slow-growing) and not life threatening. However, it can progress to involve lymph nodes, blood, and visceral (internal) organs.

Types include:

> Mycosis fungoides (MF) and Sézary syndrome (SS)

> Primary cutaneous CD30+ T-cell lymphoproliferative disorders (PCLPDs)

The most common types of CTCL are mycosis fungoides and Sézary syndrome.

PCLPDs include primary cutaneous anaplastic large cell lymphoma (PC-ALCL), lymphomatoid papulosis (LyP), and "borderline" cases with overlapping features.

About this book

This book will discuss treatment options for the following:

> Primary cutaneous marginal zone lymphoma (PCMZL)

> Primary cutaneous follicle center lymphoma (PCFCL)

> Primary cutaneous CD30+ T-cell lymphoproliferative disorders (PCLPDs)

More information on mycosis fungoides and Sézary syndrome can be found at NCCN.org/patientguidelines.

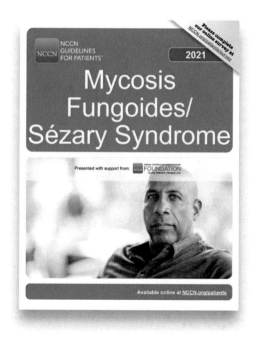

Review

> The lymphatic or lymph system is a network of tissues and organs that helps your body fight infections and disease. It is part of the immune system.

> Lymphoma is a broad term for cancer that begins in a type of white blood cell called a lymphocyte. Lymphocytes fight infections.

> Primary cutaneous lymphomas (PCLs) are a rare group of non-Hodgkin lymphomas (NHLs) found in the skin. It is not skin cancer.

> NHL is a large group of cancers divided into fast-growing (aggressive) and slow-growing (indolent) types. NHL can be formed from B-cell, T-cell, or NK-cell lymphocytes.

> PCLs can be a result of abnormal B cells, T cells, or NK cells.

> Cutaneous B-cell lymphomas (CBCLs) appear as lumps that look like small pimples called papules.

> Cutaneous T-cell lymphomas (CTCLs) appear as an itchy, red rash that can thicken or form a tumor.

Those with primary cutaneous lymphoma should be treated at centers experienced in this type of cancer.

2
Testing for PCL

13   Test results

14   General health tests

15   Skin exam

17   Blood tests

18   Imaging tests

18   Biopsy

19   Tissue tests

20   Molecular tests

22   TNM scores

24   Review

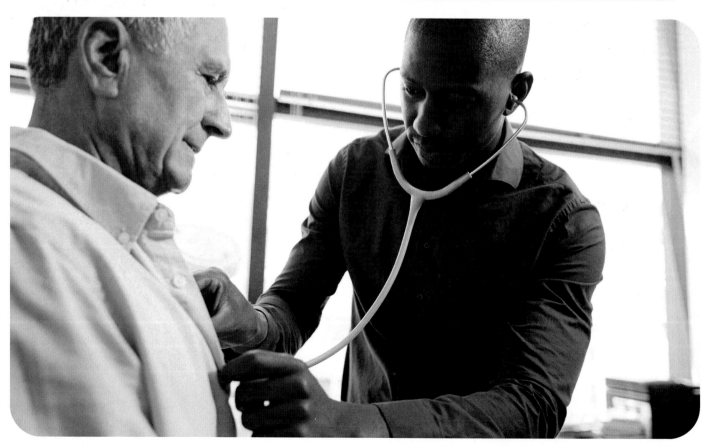

Treatment planning starts with testing. Accurate testing is needed to diagnose and treat primary cutaneous lymphomas. A biopsy is recommended before starting treatment. This chapter presents an overview of the tests you might receive and what to expect.

Test results

Results from blood and tissue tests, imaging studies, and biopsy will determine your treatment plan. It is important you understand what these tests mean. Ask questions and keep copies of your test results. Online patient portals are a great way to access your test results.

Whether you are going for a second opinion, test, or office visit, keep these things in mind:

> Bring someone with you to doctor visits, if possible.

> Write down questions and take notes during appointments. Don't be afraid to ask your care team questions. Get to know your care team and let them get to know you.

> Get copies of blood tests, imaging results, and reports about the specific type of cancer you have. It will be helpful when getting a second opinion.

> Organize your papers. Create files for insurance forms, medical records, and test results. You can do the same on your computer.

> Keep a list of contact information for everyone on your care team. Add it to your binder or notebook. Hang the list on your fridge or keep it by the phone.

Create a medical binder

A medical binder or notebook is a great way to organize all of your records in one place.

• Make copies of blood tests, imaging results, and reports about your specific type of cancer. It will be helpful when getting a second opinion.

• Choose a binder that meets your needs. Consider a zipper pocket to include a pen, small calendar, and insurance cards.

• Create folders for insurance forms, medical records, and tests results. You can do the same on your computer.

• Use online patient portals to view your test results and other records. Download or print the records to add to your binder.

• Organize your binder in a way that works for you. Add a section for questions and to take notes.

• Bring your medical binder to appointments. You never know when you might need it!

General health tests

Medical history

A medical history is a record of all health issues and treatments you have had in your life. Be prepared to list any illness or injury and when it happened. Bring a list of old and new medicines and any over-the-counter medicines, herbals, or supplements you take. Tell your doctor about any symptoms you have. A medical history will help determine which treatment is best for you.

Family history

Some cancers and other diseases can run in families. Your doctor will ask about the health history of family members who are blood relatives. This information is called a family history. Ask family members about their health issues like heart disease, cancer, and diabetes, and at what age they were diagnosed.

Physical exam

During a physical exam, a health care provider may:

> Check your temperature, blood pressure, pulse, and breathing rate

> Weigh you

> Listen to your lungs and heart

> Look in your eyes, ears, nose, and throat

> Feel and apply pressure to parts of your body to see if organs are of normal size, are soft or hard, or cause pain when touched. Tell your doctor if you feel pain.

> Feel for enlarged lymph nodes in your neck, underarm, and groin. Tell the doctor if you have felt any lumps or have any pain.

> Conduct a complete skin exam

Doctors should perform a thorough physical exam, including skim exam, with a complete health history.

The skin

Primary cutaneous lymphomas (PCLs) develop in skin and can look like a rash, lumps, bumps, or tumor.

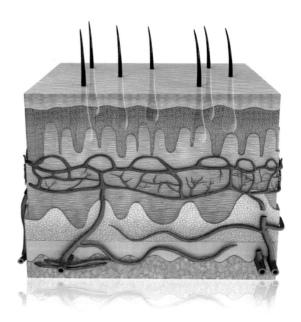

Skin exam

It is important to find an experienced dermatologist to conduct a skin exam. A complete skin exam looks for signs of PCL. PCL might appear as a rash, lumps, bumps, or tumor. A rash is an area of irritated or swollen skin. Many rashes are itchy, red, painful, and irritated. As a rash, PCL might come and go. This doesn't mean the cancer is cured.

The amount of cancer is measured using the size of your hand. One hand is equal to 1 percent (1%) of your total body surface area (BSA). In addition, any tumors will be measured by their depth, height, size, and region of the body. Keeping a photo journal might help track your skin changes over time.

The skin

Skin is the largest organ in your body. Not only does it protect your body, but it tells doctors a lot about your health. Doctors take your pulse and blood pressure through your skin. They listen to your heart and lungs through your skin. They notice if the skin feels warm, hot, or cool to the touch. They can tell if maybe you aren't getting enough oxygen based on the color of your skin. Pallor is another term for pale or grayish skin that is not receiving enough oxygen.

A skin lesion is a change in color or texture. Skin lesions can appear anywhere on the body, but are most common on the lower abdomen, upper thighs, buttocks, and breasts. Some words to describe skin lesions might include patch, papule, plaque, nodule, or tumor.

Skin lesions

A papule is a very small, solid bump. A plaque is a raised or hardened lesion that forms on the skin, larger than a papule. Plaques sometimes become tumors on the skin.

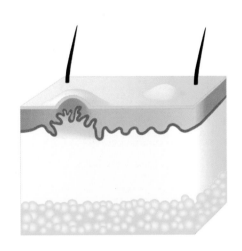

Papule

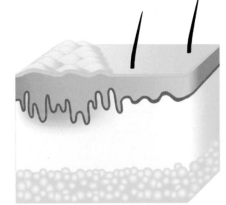

Plaque

Patch

A patch is a flat, thin, pink or red lesion of any size that forms on the skin. Patches may be dry, scaly, and itchy, and may look like eczema or psoriasis. They can be lighter than surrounding skin or brown in people with darker skin. The patches may sometimes become plaques (hard, raised lesions) on the skin.

Papule

A papule is a very small, solid lump that might look like a very small pimple. Usually papules are found in groups. Papules may be red, purple, brown, or pink.

Plaque

A plaque is a raised (elevated) or hardened (indurated) lesion of any size that forms on the skin. Plaques may be red, scaly, and itchy, and may look like eczema or psoriasis. Plaques sometimes become tumors on the skin.

Papulonodular

Papulonodular is a combination of papules and nodules found on the skin. Nodules are more raised than papules.

Tumor

A tumor is a firm, dome-shaped mass at least 1 centimeter in size.

Ulcer

A skin ulcer is an open sore or wound on the skin caused by poor blood flow.

> Keeping a photo journal might help track your skin changes over time.

Skin color

Melanin gives your skin color. Skin color is based on the amount of melanin in your skin, and the amount of oxygen and hemoglobin in your blood. Hemoglobin is a protein found inside red blood cells. Testing for the amount of hemoglobin in the blood is usually part of a complete blood count (CBC) test.

You know your skin better than anyone. Tell your doctor about your normal skin color. Show your doctor the differences in where the skin looks normal and different to you. Describe any changes. Does the area itch or burn? Is it dry? Is it red or warm to the touch? Are there bumps or a raised, smooth area? Is there an odor? Share any photos.

Blood tests

Blood tests check for signs of disease and how well organs are working. They require a sample of your blood, which is removed through a needle placed into your vein.

Complete blood count

A complete blood count (CBC) measures the levels of red blood cells (RBCs), white blood cells (WBCs), and platelets in your blood. Your doctor will want to know if you have enough RBCs to carry oxygen throughout your body, WBCs to fight infection, and platelets to control bleeding.

Comprehensive metabolic panel

A comprehensive metabolic panel (CMP) measures 14 different substances in your blood. It is usually done on the plasma part of your blood. A CMP provides important information about how well your kidneys and liver are working, among other things.

Differential

There are 5 types of WBCs: neutrophils, lymphocytes, monocytes, eosinophils, and basophils. A differential counts the number of each type of WBC. It also checks if the counts are in balance with each other.

Hepatitis B and C

Hepatitis is a virus that causes inflammation of the liver. Hepatitis B (HBV) and hepatitis C (HCV) are spread by contact with blood and other bodily fluids. A blood test will show if you had hepatitis in the past or if you have it today. Treatment with immunotherapy and chemotherapy might cause HBV to reactivate, which can cause liver damage.

HIV

Human immunodeficiency virus (HIV) causes acquired immunodeficiency syndrome (AIDS). An HIV antibody test checks for HIV antibodies in a sample of blood, urine, or saliva.

HTLV

Human T-lymphotropic virus (HTLV) testing is used to detect an infection by HTLV-I or HTLV-II. A blood test is used to detect an HTLV infection that could be the cause of a T-cell lymphoma. In the United States, all donated blood is screened for HTLV.

Lactic acid

Lactate dehydrogenase (LDH) or lactic acid dehydrogenase is an enzyme found in most cells. Dying cells release LDH into blood. Fast-growing cells, such as tumor cells, also release LDH.

Pregnancy test

If planned treatment might affect pregnancy, then those who can become pregnant will be given a pregnancy test before treatment begins.

SPEP

Serum protein electrophoresis (SPEP) examines specific proteins in the blood called globulins, which may be increased in certain conditions such as multiple myeloma.

Imaging tests

Imaging tests take pictures (images) of the inside of your body. These tests are used to look for cancer in organs and areas outside of the blood. A radiologist, an expert in test images, will write a report and send this report to your doctor. Your doctor will discuss the results with you.

X-ray

An x-ray is a type of radiation. In small doses, it is used to make pictures of the inside of the body. It might be referred to as a radiograph.

CT scan

A computed tomography (CT or CAT) scan uses x-rays and computer technology to take pictures of the inside of the body. It takes many x-rays of the same body part from different angles. All the images are combined to make one detailed picture. In most cases, contrast will be used. Contrast materials are not dyes, but substances that help certain areas in the body stand out. They are used to make the pictures clearer. Contrast materials are not permanent and will leave the body in your urine.

Tell your doctors if you have had bad reactions to contrast in the past. This is important. You might be given medicines, such as Benadryl® and prednisone, for an allergy to contrast. Contrast might not be used if you have a serious allergy or if your kidneys aren't working well.

MRI scan

A magnetic resonance imaging (MRI) scan uses radio waves and powerful magnets to take pictures of the inside of the body. It does not use x-rays. Contrast might be used.

PET scan

A positron emission tomography (PET) scan uses a radioactive drug called a tracer. A tracer is a substance injected into a vein to see where it is in the body and if it is using sugar to grow. Cancer cells show up as bright spots on PET scans. Not all bright spots are cancer. It is normal for the brain, heart, kidneys, and bladder to be bright on PET. When a PET scan is combined with CT, it is called a PET/CT scan.

Biopsy

A biopsy is the removal of a sample tissue or a group of cells for testing. It is an important part of an accurate diagnosis. Your sample should be reviewed by a pathologist who is an expert in the diagnosis of PCL. The pathologist will note the overall appearance and the size, shape, and type of your cells. This review is often referred to as histology or histopathology review. Tests will be done on the biopsied cells.

Skin lesion biopsy

A sample of your lesion will be removed and tested to confirm the type of PCL. A skin lesion biopsy can be incisional or excisional. An incisional biopsy removes an area of skin using a scalpel blade. Stitches are usually required after an incisional biopsy. An excisional biopsy removes a larger area of skin, tumor, or lesion.

Skin punch biopsy

In a skin punch biopsy, a small sample of skin and connective tissue are removed using a hand-held tool. Stitches are often used to close the opening in the skin.

Skin shave biopsy

A skin shave biopsy removes a shaving of the top layer of skin using a tool like a razor. This type of biopsy may not be recommended because it doesn't take a deep enough sample. Abnormal lymphocytes are often found under the surface of the skin.

Lymph node biopsy

A lymph node might be biopsied if cancer is suspected based on a test or physical exam. Lymph nodes are usually too small to be seen or felt. Sometimes, lymph nodes can feel swollen, enlarged, hard to the touch, or don't move when pushed (fixed or immobile). A lymph node biopsy can be done using a needle biopsy procedure or as a small surgery to remove a lymph node.

Bone marrow tests

Bone marrow tests might be done in certain cases.

There are 2 types of bone marrow tests that are often done at the same time:

> Bone marrow aspirate

> Bone marrow biopsy

Your bone marrow is like a sponge holding liquid and cells. An aspirate takes some of the liquid and cells out of the sponge, and a biopsy takes a piece of the sponge.

The samples are usually taken from the back of the hip bone (pelvis). You will likely lie on your belly or side. Your doctors will first clean and give sedation or numb your skin and outer surface of your bone. For an aspirate, a hollow needle will be pushed through your skin and into the bone. Liquid bone marrow will then be drawn into a syringe. For the biopsy, a wider needle will be used to remove a core sample. You may feel bone pain at your hip for a few days. Your skin may bruise.

Tissue tests

Tissue and cells removed during a skin biopsy will be tested.

Immunophenotyping

Immunophenotyping is a process that uses antibodies to detect the presence or absence of certain antigens. Antigens are proteins or markers that can be found on the surface of or inside white blood cells. Specific groupings of antigens are normal. However, some specific patterns of antigens are found on abnormal cells.

Immunophenotyping can be done using flow cytometry or immunohistochemistry. Flow cytometry immunophenotyping may be used to help diagnose and treat PCL. Immunophenotype can change as cancer progresses.

Flow cytometry

Flow cytometry is a laboratory method used to detect, identify, and count specific cells. Flow cytometry involves adding a light-sensitive dye to cells. The dyed cells are passed through a beam of light in a machine. The machine measures the number of cells, things like the size and shape of the cells, and proteins on the surface of thousands of cells. Flow cytometry may be used on cells from circulating (peripheral) blood, bone marrow, or a biopsy. The most common use of flow cytometry is in the identification of markers on cells, particularly in the immune system (called immunophenotyping).

Immunohistochemistry

Immunohistochemistry (IHC) is a special staining process that involves adding a chemical marker to immune cells. The cells are then studied using a microscope. IHC looks for the immunophenotype of cells from a skin biopsy. IHC panel of skin biopsy should include testing for CD3, CD4, CD8, CD10, CD20, CD30, CD56, ALK, BCL2, BCL6, IRF4/MUM1, and others.

Molecular tests

Molecular tests are used to learn more about your type of PCL and to target treatment. Talk to your care team and/or a genetic counselor about your family history of cancer.

Inside our cells are deoxyribonucleic acid (DNA) molecules. These molecules are tightly packaged into what is called a chromosome. Chromosomes contain most of the genetic information in a cell. Normal human cells contain 23 pairs of chromosomes for a total of 46 chromosomes. Each chromosome contains thousands of genes. Genes are coded instructions for the proteins your cells make. A mutation is when something goes wrong in the genetic code.

There are different types of genetic tests; some are done on molecules or proteins, some on genes, and some on chromosomes. Genetic testing might include cytogenetics or molecular testing. Cytogenetics is the study of chromosomes. Cytogenetics involves testing samples of blood, tissue, and bone marrow to look for broken, missing, rearranged, or extra chromosomes. Molecular or biomarker testing looks for specific proteins or molecules. Genes are written like this: *ALK*. Proteins are written like this: ALK.

Gene rearrangements

In gene rearrangements, part of a gene has broken off and attached to another gene. When one cell divides many times, the entire group of cells is called clonal or clonality. In clonal rearrangements, abnormal groups are found.

Molecular testing (analysis) is used to detect B-cell or T-cell rearrangements commonly found in PCL. This information can be helpful when diagnosing and treating PCL.

Examples include:

> Clonal T-cell antigen receptor *(TCR)* gene rearrangements

> Immunoglobulin heavy *(IgH)* gene rearrangement

> Anaplastic lymphoma kinase (*ALK*) gene rearrangement can be found in a subset of CD30-positive anaplastic large cell lymphomas (ALCLs). *ALK* is a gene that tells your body how to make proteins that help cells talk to each other.

> *DUSP22-IRF4* gene rearrangement is used to detect ALK-negative ALCL and a subtype of lymphomatoid papulosis (LyP)

> *TP63* rearrangement is used to define a subset of ALK-negative ALCL cases

Comparative genomic hybridization

Comparative genomic hybridization (CGH) is a technique that compares DNA samples from normal tissue and tumor tissue. It is used to detect abnormal chromosomes.

High-throughput sequencing

High-throughput sequencing (HTS) is capable of sequencing hundreds of millions of DNA molecules at a time.

Next-generation sequencing

Next-generation sequencing (NGS) is a high-throughput method used to determine a portion of a person's DNA sequence.

Karyotype

A karyotype is a picture of chromosomes. It is produced in about a week at a special lab. Doctors look for whether 46 chromosomes or 23 pairs are present. They also look for extra, missing, rearranged, or abnormal pieces of chromosomes. Since a karyotype requires growing cells, a sample of bone marrow must be used.

FISH

Fluorescence in situ hybridization (FISH) is a method that involves special dyes called probes that attach to pieces of DNA. Since this test doesn't need growing cells, it can be performed on either a bone marrow or blood sample. However, FISH can only be used for known changes. It cannot detect all the possible changes found with a karyotype. For example, FISH is used to detect *TP63* gene rearrangements by attaching probes to *TP63* (3q28) and *TBL1XR1/TP63.*

Doctors can also look for other translocations that are too small to be seen with other methods. A translocation occurs when parts of two chromosomes switch with one another.

PCR

A polymerase chain reaction (PCR) is a lab process that can make millions or billions of copies of your DNA (genetic information) in just a few hours, but results can take days. PCR is very sensitive. It can find 1 abnormal cell among more than 100,000 normal cells. These copies, called PCR product, might be used for HTS or NGS.

TNM scores

The tumor, node, metastasis (TNM) system is used to stage many cancers. In this system, the letters T, N, and M describe different areas of cancer growth. Based on biopsy and other test results, your doctor will assign a score or number to each letter. The higher the number, the larger the tumor or the more the cancer has spread to lymph nodes or other organs. A TNM example might look like this: T1N0M0 or T1, N0, M0.

> **T is for skin** – Tumor refers to size, type, and number of tumors or lesions covering the skin.

> **Node is for lymph node** – Cancer can spread to lymph nodes.

> **M is for metastasis** – Cancer can spread to distant parts of the body.

Cancer staging is often done twice.

> **Clinical stage (c)** is the rating given before any treatment. It is based on a physical exam, biopsy, and other tests.

> **Pathologic stage (p)** or surgical stage is determined by examining tissue removed during surgery such as in the removal of a lymph node. Pathologic features include size, shape, and type of cell.

The following TNM sections describe staging for PCL other than mycosis fungoides (MF) and Sézary syndrome (SS). More information on MF/SS can be found at NCCN.org/patientguidelines.

T = Skin

Lesions or tumors will be measured by their depth, height, size, and region of the body. Lesions are often measured in centimeters (cm). Body regions are based on regional lymph node drainage patterns. Body regions include head/neck, chest, upper arm, lower arm and hand, abdomen and genitals, upper leg, lower leg and feet, upper back, lower back and buttocks.

> **T1** – Solitary skin involvement

  · **T1a** is one lesion less than 5 cm

  · **T1b** is one lesion greater than 5 cm

> **T2** – Regional skin involvement with multiple lesions limited to 1 body region or 2 continuous body regions

  · **T2a** is disease limited to smaller than a 15-cm area

  · **T2b** is disease limited to a 15-cm to 20-cm area

  · **T2c** is disease in a larger than 30-cm area

> **T3** – Generalized skin involvement

  · **T3a** is multiple lesions involving 2 body regions not next to one another

  · **T3b** is multiple lesions involving 3 or more body regions

N = Node

There are hundreds of lymph nodes throughout your body. Lymph nodes work as filters to help fight infection and remove harmful things. Lymph node regions are based on the Ann Arbor Staging System. Peripheral sites include antecubital, cervical, supraclavicular, axillary, inguinal-femoral, and popliteal. Central sites include mediastinal, pulmonary hilar, paraortic, and iliac.

> **N0** means no cancer found in lymph nodes

> **N1** means involvement of 1 peripheral lymph node region that drains an area of current or prior skin involvement

> **N2** means involvement of 2 or more peripheral lymph node regions or involvement of any lymph node region that does not drain an area of current or prior skin involvement

> **N3** means cancer is found in central lymph nodes

M = Metastasis

Cancer that has spread to distant parts of the body is called metastatic. Cancer can metastasize to organs like the liver or spleen. It may be referred to as extracutaneous.

> M0 means no cancer is found in organs

> M1 means cancer is found in organs

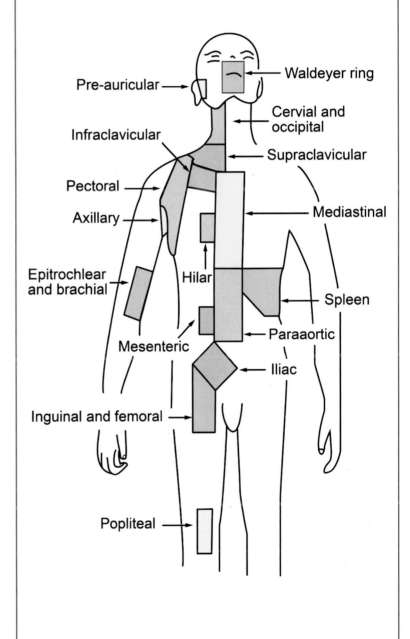

Lymph node regions

Lymph node regions based on the Ann Arbor Staging System.

https://commons.wikimedia.org/wiki/File:Lymph_node_regions.svg

- Pre-auricular
- Waldeyer ring
- Cervial and occipital
- Infraclavicular
- Supraclavicular
- Pectoral
- Mediastinal
- Axillary
- Epitrochlear and brachial
- Hilar
- Spleen
- Mesenteric
- Paraaortic
- Iliac
- Inguinal and femoral
- Popliteal

Review

> Tests are used to plan treatment and check how well treatment is working.

> Online portals are a great way to access your test results.

> Skin lesions can appear anywhere on the body, but are most common on the lower abdomen, upper thighs, buttocks, and breasts. Lesions may look like papules, patches, plaques, or nodules.

> A skin biopsy is needed to diagnose primary cutaneous lymphoma (PCL). Your sample should be reviewed by a pathologist who is an expert in the diagnosis of PCL.

> A sample from your biopsy will be tested to look for biomarkers or proteins.

> The tumor, node, metastasis (TNM) system might be used to describe your cancer.

Tell your doctor about any medicines, vitamins, over-the-counter drugs, herbals, or supplements you are taking.

3
Treating PCL

26 Multidisciplinary team

27 Surgery

27 Skin-directed therapy

28 Radiation therapy

29 Systemic therapy

30 Clinical trials

31 Supportive care

31 Pregnancy and fertility

32 Review

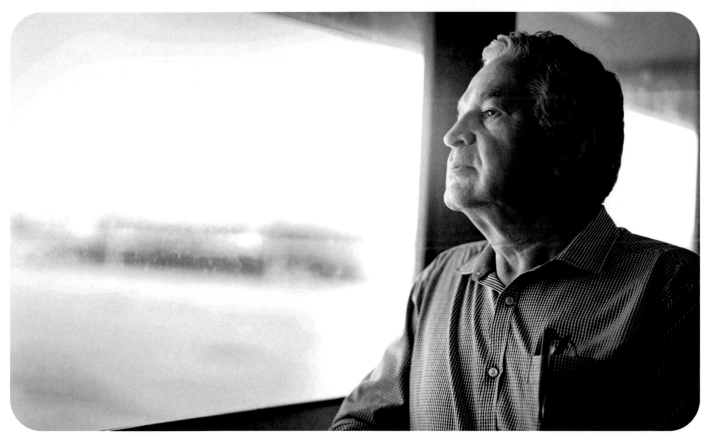

This chapter presents an overview of the types of treatment for PCL and what to expect. Together, you and your doctor will choose a treatment plan that is right for you.

Multidisciplinary team

Those with primary cutaneous lymphoma (PCL) should seek treatment or consultation at centers with expertise in the management of PCL.

Treating PCL takes a team approach. Treatment decisions should involve a multidisciplinary team (MDT) or a team of doctors from different fields of medicine who have knowledge (expertise) and experience with your type of cancer. This is important. Ask who will coordinate your care.

Possible members of the MDT:

> A dermatologist specializes in the diagnosis and treatment of skin diseases.

> A hematologist/oncologist specializes in blood diseases and cancers and their treatment.

> A pathologist interprets the cells and tissues removed during a biopsy or surgery and performs flow cytometry, immunohistochemistry, and genetic studies.

> A radiation oncologist prescribes and plans radiation therapy to treat cancer.

> A radiologist interprets the results of x-rays and other imaging tests.

Depending on your type of care, the team might include:

> A gastroenterologist who diagnoses and treats disorders of the digestive system

> A general surgeon who has specialized knowledge and experience related to the diagnosis, preoperative, operative, and postoperative care for the whole patient

> An interventional radiologist who performs needle biopsies, ablation therapies, and embolizations, and places ports for treatment

> A plastic surgeon who performs operations to improve function or reconstruct missing areas

> A vascular surgeon who specializes in procedures involving arteries, veins, and lymph circulation

Some members of your care team will be with you throughout cancer treatment, while others will only be there for parts of it. Get to know your care team and let them get to know you.

Keep a list of names and contact information for each member of your team. This will make it easier for you and anyone involved in your care to know whom to contact with questions or concerns.

You know your body better than anyone. Help other team members understand:

> How you feel

> What you need

> What is working and what is not

> Your goals for treatment

Surgery

Surgery is an operation or procedure to remove a lesion or tumor from the body. The type of surgery you receive depends on size, location, and number of tumors. It is also called excision or excisional surgery. The usual role for surgery is to biopsy suspicious lesions, not to totally remove (excise) the lymphoma.

Skin-directed therapy

Types of therapy focused on the skin include topical therapy, local radiation, and phototherapy.

Topical therapy
Topical treatments are put on the surface of the skin. It might be a lotion, gel, or ointment. Types of topical therapy are described next.

Topical and intralesional corticosteroids
Steroid is the short name for corticosteroid. Steroids are man-made and are used to reduce inflammation. Steroids used to treat PCL can be topical or intralesional. An intralesional steroid is injected directly into a lesion on or immediately below the skin.

Steroids can cause short-term and long-term side effects. Ask your care team about possible side effects. Corticosteroids are not the same as the steroids used by some athletes.

Topical nitrogen mustard
Nitrogen mustard (mechlorethamine hydrochloride) stops or slows the growth of cancer.

Topical retinoids
Retinoids are products related to vitamin A. Topical bexarotene (Targretin® gel) and topical tazarotene (Tazorac® Gel, Tazorac® Cream) are retinoids applied to the skin to treat lesions.

Topical carmustine
Carmustine is a chemotherapy that stops or slows the growth of cancer. Topical carmustine (BiCNU®) is applied to lesions.

Topical imiquimod
Topical imiquimod is used to treat certain types of flat, scaly growths on the skin. Brand names include Aldara® and Zyclara®.

Local radiation
Local radiation treats the skin lesion only. Involved-site radiation therapy (ISRT) is a type of local radiation. It can be used on lymph nodes and/or skin lesions. The type of radiation is usually electrons.

Phototherapy

Phototherapy uses different ultraviolet (UV) light wavelengths to treat skin lesions or tumors.

Types include:

> Ultraviolet light B (UVB) – exposes the skin to an artificial UVB light source for a set length of time on a regular schedule.

> Narrowband ultraviolet light B (NB-UVB) – uses a very specific UV wavelength.

> Photochemotherapy ultraviolet light A (PUVA) – combines psoralen (P) with UVA. Psoralen is a type of medicine taken by mouth (orally) that causes your skin to be sensitive to light. After taking psoralen, the skin is exposed to long-wave UV light.

> Ultraviolet light A1 (UVA1) - penetrates deep into the skin causing T cells to die.

UV can increase your risk of some skin cancers. Phototherapy may not be favored in those with a history of squamoproliferative skin neoplasms, basal cell carcinomas, or who have had melanoma.

Radiation therapy

Radiation therapy (RT) uses high-energy radiation from x-rays, photons, electrons, and other sources to kill cancer cells and shrink tumors. RT can be given alone or with other treatments. Treatment may focus on individual tumors, a small area/region of the body, the entire surface of the skin, or specific lymph nodes. RT may be used as supportive care or palliative care to help ease pain or discomfort caused by cancer.

EBRT

External beam radiation therapy (EBRT) uses a machine outside of the body to aim radiation at the tumor(s) or areas of the body.

Common types of EBRT that may be used to treat your cancer include:

> Involved-site radiation therapy (ISRT) targets a specific area of skin. It can also be used to treat specific lymph nodes with cancer.

> Total skin electron beam therapy (TSEBT) treats the entire skin surface. You might stand on a rotating platform to receive this treatment.

Less common types of EBRT that may be used to treat your cancer include:

> Three-dimensional conformal radiation therapy (3D-CRT) uses computer software and CT images to aim beams that match the shape of the tumor.

> Intensity-modulated radiation therapy (IMRT) uses small beams of different strengths to match the shape of the tumor.

> Stereotactic body radiation therapy (SBRT) uses high-energy radiation beams to treat cancers in five or fewer treatments.

> Stereotactic radiosurgery (SRS) uses special equipment to position the body and give one precise, large dose of radiation.

> Particle beam RT uses protons, carbon ions, or other heavy ions to treat cancer.

Systemic therapy

Systemic therapy works throughout the body. It includes retinoids, chemotherapy, targeted therapy, and immunotherapy. Systemic therapy might be used alone or with other therapies.

Chemotherapy

Chemotherapy kills fast-growing cells throughout the body, including cancer cells and normal cells. All chemotherapies affect the instructions (genes) that tell cancer cells how and when to grow and divide. There are many chemotherapies used to treat primary cutaneous lymphomas.

Targeted therapy

Targeted therapy focuses on specific or unique features of cancer cells. Targeted therapies seek out how cancer cells grow, divide, and move in the body. These drugs stop the action of molecules that help cancer cells grow and/or survive.

Immunotherapy

Immunotherapy is a targeted therapy that increases the activity of your immune system. By doing so, it improves your body's ability to find and destroy cancer cells. Immunotherapy can be given alone or with other types of treatment.

Retinoids

Retinoids are products related to vitamin A, but can stop the growth of cancer cells. When taken by mouth (orally), they work throughout the body.

Did you know?

The terms "chemotherapy" and "systemic therapy" are often used interchangeably, but they are not the same. Chemotherapy, targeted therapy, and immunotherapy are all types of systemic therapy.

Warnings!

You might be asked to stop taking or avoid certain herbal supplements when on a systemic therapy. Some supplements can affect the ability of a drug to do its job. This is called a drug interaction. It is critical to speak with your care team about any supplements you may be taking.

Some examples include:

> Turmeric

> Gingko biloba

> Green tea extract

> St. John's Wort

Certain medicines can also affect the ability of a drug to do its job. Antacids, heart medicine, and antidepressants are just some of the medicines that might interact with a systemic therapy. This is why it is important to tell your doctor about any medications, vitamins, over-the-counter (OTC) drugs, herbals, or supplements you are taking. **Bring a list with you to every visit.**

Clinical trials

Clinical trials study how safe and helpful tests and treatments are for people. Clinical trials find out how to prevent, diagnose, and treat a disease like cancer. Because of clinical trials, scientists and doctors have found, and are continuing to find, new and effective therapies in the management of cancer.

Clinical trials have 4 phases.

> **Phase I trials** aim to find the safest and best dose of a new drug. Another aim is to find the best way to give the drug with the fewest side effects.

> **Phase II trials** assess if a drug works for a specific type of cancer.

> **Phase III trials** formally and scientifically compare a new drug to a standard treatment.

> **Phase IV trials** evaluate a drug's longer term safety and treatment results after it has been approved.

To join a clinical trial, you must meet the conditions of the study. Patients in a clinical trial often are alike in terms of their cancer and general health. This helps to ensure that any change is from the treatment and not because of differences between patients.

If you decide to join a clinical trial, you will need to review and sign a paper called an informed consent form. This form describes the study in detail, including the risks and benefits. Even after you sign a consent form, you can stop taking part in a clinical trial at any time.

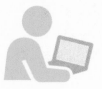

Finding a clinical trial

In the United States

NCCN Cancer Centers
NCCN.org/cancercenters

The National Cancer Institute (NCI)
cancer.gov/about-cancer/treatment/clinical-trials/search

Worldwide

The U.S. National Library of Medicine (NLM)
clinicaltrials.gov/

Need help finding a clinical trial?
NCI's Cancer Information Service (CIS)

1.800.4.CANCER (1.800.422.6237)

cancer.gov/contact

Ask your treatment team if there is an open clinical trial that you can join. There may be clinical trials where you're getting treatment or at other treatment centers nearby. Discuss the risks and benefits of joining a clinical trial with your care team. Together, decide if a clinical trial is right for you.

Supportive care

Supportive care is health care that relieves symptoms caused by cancer or its treatment and improves quality of life. It might include pain relief (palliative care), emotional or spiritual support, financial aid, or family counseling. Supportive care is given during all cancer stages. Tell your care team how you are feeling and about any side effects. Best supportive care is used with other treatments to improve quality of life. Best supportive care, supportive care, and palliative care are often used interchangeably.

Treatment side effects

All cancer treatments can cause unwanted health issues. Such health issues are called side effects. Side effects depend on many factors. These factors include the drug type and dose, length of treatment, and the person. Some side effects may be harmful to your health. Others may just be unpleasant. Ask for a complete list of side effects of your treatments. Also, tell your treatment team about any new or worsening symptoms. There may be ways to help you feel better. There are also ways to prevent some side effects.

Pregnancy and fertility

If planned treatment might affect pregnancy, then those who can become pregnant will be given a pregnancy test before treatment begins. Treatment can also affect fertility in both sexes. Fertility is the ability to have children. If you think you want children in the future, ask your doctor how cancer and cancer treatment might change your fertility and sexual health.

Those with ovaries

Those who can have children will have a pregnancy test before starting treatment. Cancer treatment can hurt the baby if you are or become pregnant during treatment. Therefore, birth control to prevent pregnancy during and after treatment is recommended. Hormonal birth control may not be recommended, so ask your doctor about options.

Those with testicles

Cancer and cancer treatment can damage sperm. Therefore, use contraception (birth control) to prevent pregnancy during and after cancer treatment. If you think you want children in the future, talk to your doctor now. Sperm banking is an option.

Infertility

Infertility is the complete loss of the ability to have children. The actual risk of infertility is related to your age at time of diagnosis, treatment type(s), treatment dose, and treatment length. Chemotherapy with alkylating agents has a higher risk of infertility. Sometimes, there isn't time for fertility preservation before you start treatment. Talk to your doctor about your concerns.

Review

> Treatment decisions should involve a multidisciplinary team (MDT) or a team of doctors from different fields of medicine who have knowledge (expertise) and experience with your type of cancer.

> Skin-directed therapy focuses on the skin and includes topical therapy, local radiation, and phototherapy.

> Systemic therapy works throughout the body. It includes chemotherapy, targeted therapy, immunotherapy, and retinoids.

> Radiation therapy (RT) uses high-energy radiation from x-rays, electrons, photons, and other sources to kill cancer cells and shrink tumors.

> Clinical trials study how safe and helpful tests and cancer treatments are for people.

> Supportive care is health care that relieves symptoms caused by cancer or its treatment and improves quality of life.

> All cancer treatments can cause unwanted health issues called side effects. You will be monitored for side effects, infection, and other treatment-related issues.

> Treatment can affect fertility in both sexes. If planned treatment might affect pregnancy, then those who can become pregnant will be given a pregnancy test before treatment begins.

Get to know your care team and let them get to know you.

4
PCBCL

34 Overview

35 Diagnosis

36 Testing

37 Treatment

40 Review

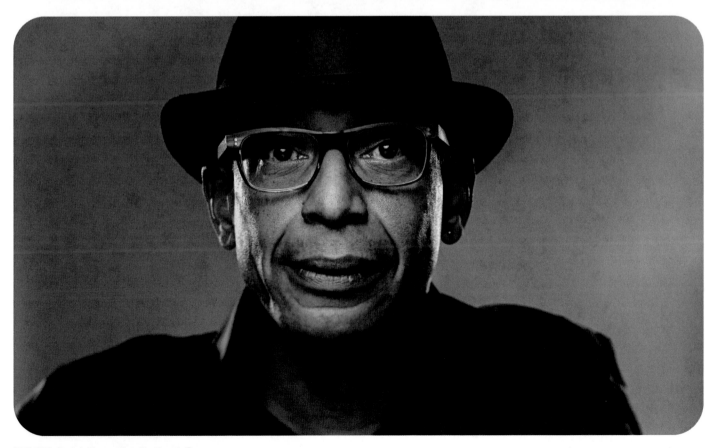

Primary cutaneous B-cell lymphoma (PCBCL) starts in B cells, a type of white blood cell. These cells make antibodies to fight infections and are an important part of the lymphatic system. This chapter is for those with primary cutaneous follicle center lymphoma (PCFCL) or primary cutaneous marginal zone lymphoma (PCMZL).

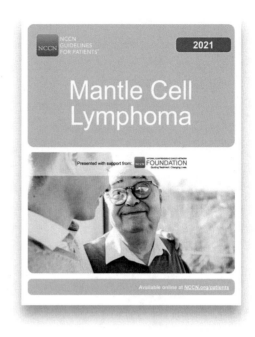

Overview

Primary cutaneous B-cell lymphoma (PCBCL or CBCL) is a rare type of cancer in which abnormal B cells (B lymphocytes) attack the skin causing nodules or lesions. Most are indolent or slow-growing.

Types include:

> Primary cutaneous follicle center lymphoma (PCFCL)

> Primary cutaneous marginal zone lymphoma (PCMZL)

> Primary cutaneous diffuse large B-cell lymphoma, leg type (PC-DLBCL, leg type)

Mantle cell lymphoma is not a PCBCL. If it is found on the skin, testing will look for disease inside the body. For more information about mantle cell lymphoma, see *NCCN Guidelines for Patients: Mantle Cell Lymphoma (MCL)* at NCCN.org/patientguidelines.

PCFCL
PCFCL (or CFCL) is generally slow-growing and most often found in the scalp and forehead. PCFCL develops slowly over months or years, and may look like a single tumor or several nodules grouped together. Tumors are pink or reddish and slightly raised and smooth. Usually, PCFCL is BCL6-positive, CD20-positive, IRF4/MUM1-negative, CD3-negative, and FOXP1-negative. Treatment for PCFCL will be discussed in this chapter.

PCMZL
PCMZL (or CMZL) is generally slow-growing and most often found in the torso and limbs. It appears as pink or red papules, nodules, and/or tumors. PCMZL is always negative for BCL6 and CD10, and often BCL2-positive. Treatment for PCMZL will be discussed in this chapter.

Primary cutaneous DLBCL, leg type
This type of DLBCL consists of large transformed B cells that typically appear as red or bluish-red tumors. Despite its name, the disease can involve the torso, arms, legs, buttocks, or anywhere on the body. These lymphomas can also spread to areas other than the skin. Treatment for PC-DLBCL, leg type is not covered in this book.

Diagnosis

A skin biopsy is an important part of diagnosis. Since it is very difficult to distinguish between PCFCL and PC-DLBCL, leg type, biopsy results should be reviewed by an expert pathologist. Immunohistochemistry (IHC) and immunophenotyping will help determine the specific type of primary cutaneous B-cell lymphoma. See Guide 1.

A cell must make a copy of its chromosomes before dividing into two cells. Sometimes, there are mistakes in the copies. One type of mistake happens when parts of two chromosomes break off and switch with each other. This is called a translocation. The t(14;18) translocation only rarely occurs in primary cutaneous B-cell lymphoma. Therefore, the detection of a t(14;18) translocation suggests the presence of systemic follicular lymphoma (FL). If FL is suspected, then you might have cytogenetic testing.

Treatment for follicular lymphoma can be found at NCCN.org/patientguidelines.

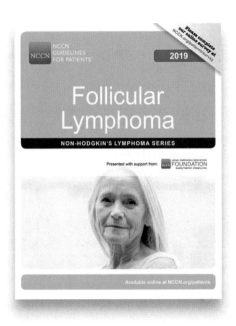

Guide 1
Diagnosis: Primary cutaneous B-cell lymphoma (PCBCL)

Needed	Biopsy of skin sites
	Biopsy review done by pathologist who is an expert in the diagnosis of primary cutaneous B-cell lymphomas
	Immunophenotyping of skin biopsy to include immunohistochemistry (IHC) panel for CD20, CD3, CD10, BCL2, BCL6, IRF4/MUM1
In some cases	IHC panel, which may include Ki-67, CD5, CD43, CD21, CD23, cyclin D1, kappa/lambda (IHC or ISH), EBER-ISH
	Assessment of IgM, IgD, and FOXP1 expression (to help distinguish PC-DLBCL, leg type from PCFCL)
	Cytogenetics (FISH and karyotype) to look for t(14;18) if systemic follicular lymphoma (FL) suspected
	Flow cytometry or *IgH* gene rearrangement studies for determining B-cell clonality

Testing

After diagnosis, further testing will be done.
These include general health, blood, and
imaging tests. For possible tests, see Guide 2.

Guide 2 Testing: PCBCL	
Needed	Medical history
	Physical exam
	Complete skin exam
	Complete blood count (CBC) with differential
	Comprehensive metabolic panel (CMP)
	Lactate dehydrogenase (LDH)
	Chest/abdomen/pelvis CT with contrast and/or PET/CT
	Pregnancy test if treatment might affect pregnancy
In some cases	Bone marrow biopsy
	Peripheral blood flow cytometry
	SPEP/quantitative immunoglobulins for PCMZL
	HIV testing
	Hepatitis B and C testing
	Discussion of fertility and sperm banking, if treatment might affect fertility

Treatment

This section discusses treatment for primary cutaneous follicle center lymphoma (PCFCL) and primary cutaneous marginal zone lymphoma (PCMZL). Treatment is based the number of skin lesions and their location. Disease may be solitary, regional, generalized skin only, or generalized extracutaneous. At the end of treatment, imaging tests are needed to assess response. PET/CT (strongly preferred) or chest/abdomen/pelvis CT with contrast are recommended. For treatment options, see Guide 3.

Guide 3
Treatment options: PCBCL

Solitary (T1) or regional (T2)	Local ISRT (preferred) and/or excision
	In some cases: • Observation • Skin-directed therapies • Intralesional steroids
Generalized skin diease (T3)	• Observation • Skin-directed therapies • Local ISRT • Intralesional steroids • Rituximab • Other systemic therapy

Solitary or regional disease

A solitary lesion is one lesion (T1). Regional lesions can be multiple lesions limited to one body region or two adjoining regions (T2). Disease area will be measured.

Options include:

> Local ISRT (preferred) and/or excision

> In some cases, observation, skin-directed therapies, or intralesional steroids

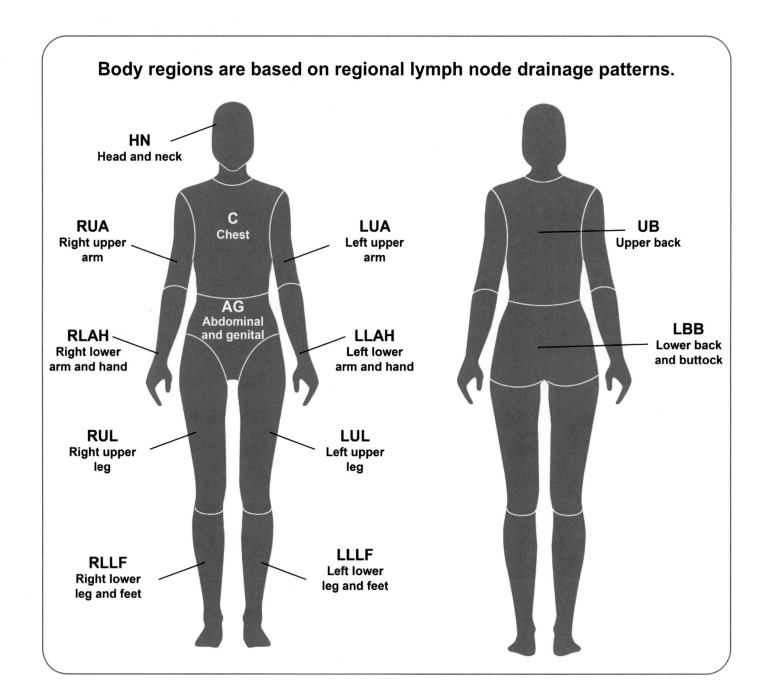

Body regions are based on regional lymph node drainage patterns.

HN Head and neck

RUA Right upper arm

C Chest

LUA Left upper arm

UB Upper back

AG Abdominal and genital

RLAH Right lower arm and hand

LLAH Left lower arm and hand

LBB Lower back and buttock

RUL Right upper leg

LUL Left upper leg

RLLF Right lower leg and feet

LLLF Left lower leg and feet

The preferred treatment is local involved-site radiation therapy (ISRT). It might be done with excision. Excision is the removal of a lesion or tumor. Other options are possible in some cases. Local ISRT is the preferred initial treatment, but not necessarily the preferred treatment for relapse. Initial treatment is the first treatment used. It might be called primary treatment.

After initial treatment, response will be assessed. You might enter a period of observation if there are no signs of disease. Relapse is cancer that returns after a disease-free period. If cancer relapses or progresses, treatment will depend on the number of lesions and regions, and whether or not there are any symptoms. Relapsed regional disease will be treated with a different option than before.

Generalized skin-only disease

Generalized skin-only disease covers a larger area of the body than regional disease. There are multiple lesions that involve 2 or more body regions (T3) not next to one another. Disease is not found in lymph nodes, blood, or other organs.

Treatment options include:

> Observation

> Skin-directed therapies

> Local ISRT

> Intralesional steroids

> Rituximab

> Other systemic therapy

Treatment targets the skin lesions. Some treatments are placed directly on or in the lesion, while others work inside the body. ISRT targets a specific area of skin. Observation or "wait-and-see" might be an option for someone without symptoms (asymptomatic). After initial treatment, response will be assessed.

For relapsed or progressive disease, treatment will be based on if disease is generalized (skin only) or extracutaneous (outside the skin).

Refractory disease does not respond to treatment. It may be resistant at the beginning of treatment or it may become resistant during treatment. If refractory disease, then treat with another therapy from the list of treatment options.

Extracutaneous disease

Extracutaneous disease is found outside the skin. This is cancer that might be found in the lymph nodes, blood, or organs. If you have PCL and later get extracutaneous disease, you will keep your original PCL diagnosis, but the stage will change.

If you have a skin lesion and testing finds extracutaneous disease, you often (but not always) would be classified as having systemic lymphoma. Treatments are based on the type of B-cell lymphoma. For example, PCFCL found inside the body will be treated as follicular lymphoma (FL).

For more information on B-cell lymphomas, see NCCN.org/patientguidelines.

Review

> Primary cutaneous B-cell lymphoma (PCBCL) starts in B cells, a type of white blood cell.

> A skin biopsy is an important part of diagnosis. Results should be reviewed by an expert pathologist.

> Immunohistochemistry (IHC) and immunophenotyping will help determine the specific type of PCBCL.

> Lesions or tumors will be measured by their depth, height, size, and region of the body. Lesions are often measured in centimeters (cm).

> Body regions are based on regional lymph node drainage patterns. Body regions include head/neck, chest, upper arm, lower arm and hand, abdomen and genitals, upper leg, lower leg and feet, upper back, lower back, and buttocks.

> Treatment is based on the number of skin lesions and their location.

> Observation or "wait-and-see" might be an option for someone without symptoms (asymptomatic).

> At the end of treatment, imaging tests are needed to assess response.

> Generalized extracutaneous disease is found outside the skin. Cancer may be in lymph nodes, blood, or internal organs such as the liver or spleen.

Local involved-site radiation therapy (ISRT) is the preferred initial treatment, but not necessarily the preferred treatment for relapse.

5

PCLPD

42 Overview

43 Diagnosis

43 Treatment

44 Review

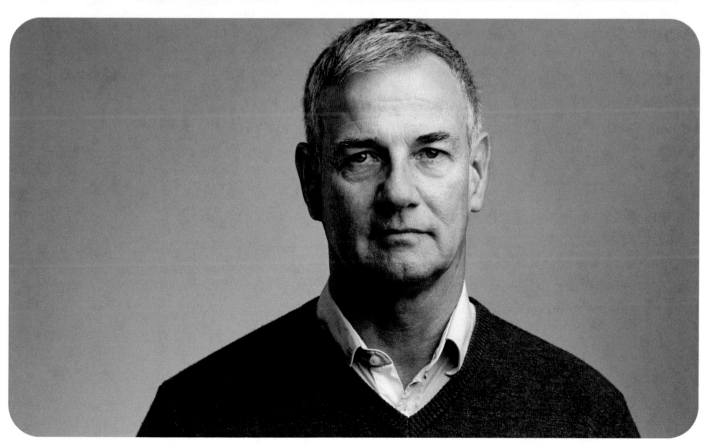

Lymphocytes of the lymphatic system grow out of control (proliferate) in lymphoproliferative disorders. In primary cutaneous CD30+ T-cell lymphoproliferative disorders (PCLPDs), T cells that are CD30-positive (CD30+) cause skin lesions or nodules. Types of PCLPD include cutaneous anaplastic large cell lymphoma (ALCL), lymphomatoid papulosis (LyP), and borderline cases.

Overview

In lymphoproliferative disorders (LPDs), a type of white blood cell called a lymphocyte grows out of control (proliferates). Primary cutaneous CD30+ T-cell lymphoproliferative disorders (PCLPDs) are a group of diseases that include lymphomatoid papulosis (LyP), cutaneous anaplastic large cell lymphoma (ALCL), and borderline cases. In PCLPD, T cells or T lymphocytes that are CD30-positive (CD30+) cause skin lesions or nodules.

Diagnosis aims to distinguish between primary cutaneous anaplastic large cell lymphoma (PC-ALCL) and LyP. The diagnosis is based on the appearance of the lesions and how the disease behaves over time (clinical course). Biopsies of both disorders will look the same!

PC-ALCL is defined by the presence of anaplastic large cells. Lesions appear on the skin as one or more raised, red lesions or nodules. LyP is a benign, chronic, recurring, self-healing condition. Papulonodular skin lesions appear on the skin as small bumps and nodules.

In addition, a person can have both PCLPD and mycosis fungoides. Mycosis fungoides is a type of primary cutaneous T-cell lymphoma.

For more information on mycosis fungoides and CD30+ transformed mycosis fungoides, see *NCCN Guidelines for Patients: Mycosis Fungoides/Sézary Syndrome at* NCCN.org/patientguidelines.

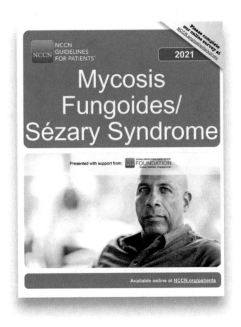

Diagnosis

An accurate diagnosis is needed to determine the type of PCLPD. Diagnosis includes a complete skin exam, a biopsy of suspicious skin sites, and immunophenotyping. Immunohistochemistry (IHC) panel will include: CD3, CD4, CD8, CD20, CD30, CD56, and ALK.

Typically, immunophenotyping shows that 75 percent (75%) or more of T cells are CD30+. This means that at least 3 out of every 4 T cells are CD30+. For diagnostic tests, see Guide 4.

Treatment

Treatment will be based on the type of PCLPD.

For treatment of

> Primary cutaneous anaplastic large cell lymphoma (PC-ALCL), see Chapter 6.

> Lymphomatoid papulosis (LyP), see Chapter 7.

Guide 4
Diagnosis: Primary Cutaneous CD30+ T-Cell Lymphoproliferative Disorders

Needed	Disease confirmation using histopathology and eliminating other causes
	Biopsy of suspicious skin sites
	Complete skin exam to look for evidence of mycosis fungoides
	Biopsy of all types (punch, incisional, or excisional) of lesions
	Biopsy review done by pathologist who is an expert in the diagnosis of cutaneous T-cell lymphomas (CTCLs)
	Immunophenoptyping using IHC on skin biopsy: • CD3, CD4, CD8, CD20, CD30, CD56, ALK
In some cases	Other IHC tests on skin biopsy: • CD2, CD5, CD7, CD25, TIA1, granzyme B, perforin, GM1, EBER-ISH, IRF4/MUM1, EMA
	Molecular analysis to detect clonal *TCR* gene rearrangements or other assessment of clonality
	FISH to detect *ALK* and *DUSP22* gene rearrangementsa
	Excisional or incisional biopsy of suspicious lymph nodes
	Assessment of HTLV-1 serology

Review

> In lymphoproliferative disorders (LPDs), cells of the lymphatic system called lymphocytes grow out of control (proliferate).

> Primary cutaneous CD30+ T-cell lymphoproliferative disorders (PCLPDs) are a group of diseases that includes lymphomatoid papulosis (LyP), anaplastic large cell lymphoma (ALCL), and borderline cases.

> In PCLPD, T cells or T lymphocytes that are CD30-positive (CD30+) cause skin lesions or nodules.

> Diagnosis includes a complete skin exam, a biopsy of suspicious skin sites, and immunophenotyping. Additional tests might be performed.

> Diagnosis aims to distinguish between ALCL and LyP.

> A person can have both PCLPD and mycosis fungoides.

In primary cutaneous CD30+ T-cell lymphoproliferative disorders (PCLPDs), T lymphocytes that are CD30-positive (CD30+) cause skin lesions or nodules.

6
Cutaneous ALCL

46 Overview

47 Testing

47 Primary cutaneous ALCL

49 Cutaneous ALCL with regional node

50 Review

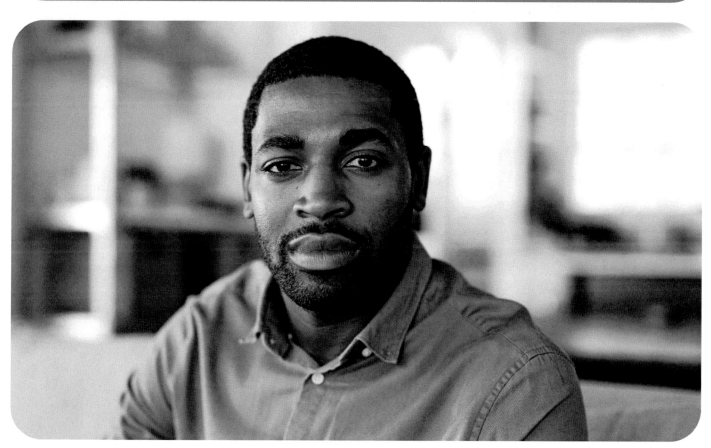

Cutaneous anaplastic large cell lymphoma (ALCL) is a type of primary cutaneous CD30+ T-cell lymphoproliferative disorder (PCLPD). Cutaneous ALCL appears in the skin as one or more raised lesions or nodules, and may be found in lymph nodes. Together, you and your doctor will choose a treatment plan that is right for you.

Overview

Anaplastic large cell lymphoma (ALCL) can be found in the skin, the lymph nodes, or in organs throughout the body. When ALCL appears in the skin, it is called primary cutaneous ALCL (PC-ALCL) or cutaneous ALCL. These words may be used interchangeably.

Cutaneous ALCL is a type of primary cutaneous CD30+ T-cell lymphoproliferative disorder (PCLPD). In PCLPD, T cells that are CD30-positive (CD30+) cause skin lesions or nodules. In PC-ALCL, lesions appear on the skin as one or more raised, red lesions or nodules. When disease is found in a nearby (regional) lymph node, it is no longer called "primary" cutaneous ALCL. It is now referred to as cutaneous ALCL. Sometimes, cutaneous ALCL can extend beyond the skin and lymph nodes to organs. If this occurs, it is usually treated like systemic ALCL.

For treatment of systemic ALCL, see *NCCN Guidelines for Patients: Peripheral T-cell Lymphoma* at NCCN.org/patientguidelines

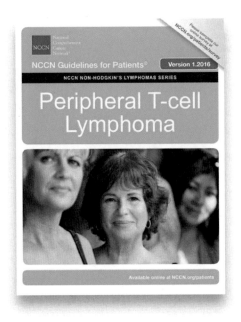

Testing

Testing will include general health, imaging, and blood tests. If cancer is suspected in a lymph node, then a lymph node biopsy will be done. A bone marrow aspiration and biopsy are possible. If planned treatment might affect pregnancy, then those who can become pregnant will be given a pregnancy test before treatment begins. Treatment can also affect fertility in both sexes. Talk to your doctor if you have concerns about your fertility.

For possible tests, see Guide 5.

Primary cutaneous ALCL

Primary cutaneous ALCL is a slowing-growing (indolent), persistent disease. Regression of lesions can occur. This means that lesions may go away (regress). Lesions often return, but seem to respond well to treatment. Not everyone responds to treatment the same way. Some respond better than expected. Others respond worse. Treatment for PC-ALCL is based on the number of lesions and their location.

Guide 5 Testing: Cutaneous ALCL	
Needed	Medical history
	Physical exam that includes applying pressure to lymph nodes, liver, and spleen
	Complete skin exam
	Complete blood count (CBC) with differential
	Comprehensive metabolic panel (CMP)
	Lactate dehydrogenase (LDH)
	Chest/abdomen/pelvis CT with contrast or whole body PET/CT (arms and legs included when needed)
	Biopsy of suspicious lymph nodes
	Bone marrow aspiration and biopsy (if needed)
In some cases	Pregnancy test if treatment might affect pregnancy
	Discussion of fertility and sperm banking, if treatment might affect fertility

One or grouped lesions

Primary treatment is the first treatment. Treatment aims to remove the lesion. This can be done using surgery (excision) and/or involved-site radiation therapy (ISRT). ISRT is more common.

After a response to treatment, you will be observed for recurrence. Recurrence or relapse is the return of one or more lesions. If a lesion returns and is confined to the skin, then you can be retreated with excision and/or ISRT. If no response or lesions seem resistant (refractory) to treatment, then you will be treated as described below in multifocal lesions.

Multifocal lesions

When there are lesions in multiple locations, primary treatment focuses on systemic therapy. A skin-directed therapy might be added. See Guide 6.

After a response to treatment, you will be observed for recurrence. Recurrence or relapse is the return of multifocal lesions. If relapse, no response, or lesions seem resistant (refractory) to treatment, then options include:

> Clinical trial

> Same treatment as before (unless refractory or intolerant)

> Different treatment from before

> Other systemic therapies

Relapsed disease often responds well to the same treatment. Partial response should be treated with the primary treatment options not yet received to improve response before moving on to treatment for refractory disease. Those with disease relapse or persistent disease after initial primary treatment may be candidates for clinical trials.

Guide 6
Primary treatment options: Multifocal lesions

Brentuximab vedotin (preferred)

Other recommended regimens with or without skin-directed therapies

Methotrexate

Systemic retinoids

Pralatrexate

Observation, if asymptomatic

Cutaneous ALCL with regional node

When disease is found in a nearby (regional) lymph node, it is referred to as cutaneous ALCL. A lymph node biopsy is needed to confirm disease.

This section describes treatment for cutaneous ALCL with regional node (N1). It does not include systemic ALCL, which is disease found throughout the body. Treatment aims to reduce the amount of skin lesions and disease in lymph nodes. Involved-site radiation therapy (ISRT) may include lymph nodes and primary skin lesions.

Primary treatment
Primary treatment is the first treatment used. See Guide 7.

Preferred treatments:

> Brentuximab vedotin with or without ISRT

> ISRT, in certain cases

Other recommended options:

> Brentuximab vedotin with CHP

> Methotrexate with or without ISRT

> Pralatrexate with or without ISRT

> CHOP or CHOEP with ISRT in some cases

Some options include multiagent chemotherapy. This is a combination of systemic therapies.

Types of multiagent chemotherapy:

> CHP (cyclophosphamide, doxorubicin, and prednisone)

> CHOP (cyclophosphamide, doxorubicin, vincristine, and prednisone)

> CHOEP (cyclophosphamide, doxorubicin, vincristine, etoposide, and prednisone)

Guide 7
Primary treatment options: Cutaneous ALCL with regional node

Preferred	• Brentuximab vedotin • Brentuximab vedotin with ISRT • ISRT in some cases
Other	• Brentuximab vedotins with CHP • Methotrexate with or without ISRT • Pralatrexate with or without ISRT • CHOP or CHOEP with or without ISRT in some cases

Relapse or refractory disease

After a response to treatment, you will be observed for recurrence. Recurrence or relapse is the return of disease. If relapse, no response, or lesions seem resistant (refractory) to treatment, then options include:

> Clinical trial

> Same treatment as before (unless refractory or intolerant)

> Different treatment from before

> Other systemic therapies

Relapsed disease often responds well to the same treatment. Partial response should be treated with the primary treatment options not yet received to improve response before moving onto treatment for refractory disease. Those with disease relapse or persistent disease after initial primary treatment may be candidates for clinical trials.

Review

> Anaplastic large cell lymphoma (ALCL) is a type of primary cutaneous CD30+ T-cell lymphoproliferative disorder (PCLPD).

> Primary cutaneous ALCL (PC-ALCL) appears in the skin as one or more raised, red lesions or nodules. Treatment is based on the number of lesions and their location.

> When disease is found in a nearby (regional) lymph node, it is referred to as cutaneous ALCL. A lymph node biopsy is needed to confirm cutaneous ALCL with regional node (N1) disease.

> Primary treatment is the first treatment.

> Relapse is disease that returns after a disease-free period. Relapsed disease often responds well to the same treatment.

> A clinical trial may be an option.

7
LyP

52   **Overview**

52   **Testing**

53   **Limited lesions**

54   **Widespread lesions**

55   **Monitoring**

55   **Review**

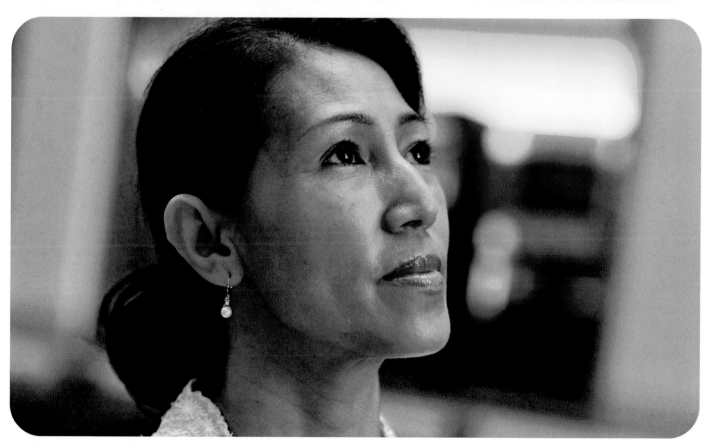

Lymphomatoid papulosis (LyP) is a benign, chronic, recurring disease of the immune system. Lesions appear on the skin as small bumps and nodules called papulonodular skin lesions.

occurs when cells of the lymphatic system grow excessively. Lymphoproliferative disorders are often treated like cancer, but they are not cancer.

Overview

Lymphomatoid papulosis (LyP) is a benign, chronic, recurring disease of the immune system. Lesions appear on the skin as small bumps and nodules called papulonodular skin lesions. These lesions are CD4+ and CD30+.

LyP is a primary cutaneous CD30+ T-cell lymphoproliferative disorder (PCLPD). An LPD

Testing

Tests will include general health, blood, and skin exam. If planned treatment might affect pregnancy, then those who can become pregnant will be given a pregnancy test before treatment begins. Treatment can also affect fertility in both sexes. Talk to your doctor if you have concerns about your fertility. For possible tests, see Guide 8.

Guide 8 Testing: Lymphomatoid papulosis (LyP)	
Needed	Medical history
	Physical exam that includes applying pressure to lymph nodes, liver, and spleen
	Complete skin exam
	Complete blood count (CBC) with differential
	Comprehensive metabolic panel (CMP)
	Lactate dehydrogenase (LDH)
In some cases	Pregnancy test if treatment might affect pregnancy
	Discussion of fertility and sperm banking, if treatment might affect fertility
	Chest/abdomen/pelvis CT with contrast or whole body PET/CT (arms and legs included when needed)
	Bone marrow aspiration and biopsy (not done for typical LyP, only done to exclude lymphoma)

Limited lesions

Without symptoms

An asymptomatic person is without symptoms. Observation is the preferred option for those with limited lesions who are asymptomatic. Topical steroids are also an option.

With symptoms

If you have limited lesions with symptoms, treatment aims to reduce symptoms. Topical steroids and phototherapy are the most commonly used skin-directed therapies for primary or initial treatment. Observation is also an option.

Response

If disease is responding to treatment, then you will continue with treatment.

If no response or refractory disease, then the options are:

> Another treatment not used before

> Other regimens

> Clinical trial

Observation is the preferred option for those who are asymptomatic.

Widespread lesions

Treatment for widespread or extensive lesions aims to reduce the number of lesions and any discomfort they may cause. This may be done using skin-directed or systemic therapies. See Guide 9.

Primary treatment options:

- Observation (preferred for asymptomatic)
- Methotrexate
- Phototherapy
- Systemic retinoids
- Topical steroids
- Topical mechlorethamine

An asymptomatic person is without symptoms. Observation is the preferred option for those who are asymptomatic.

Response

If disease is responding to treatment, then you will be observed for recurrence. Recurrence or relapse is the return of disease.

For relapse, options are:

- Clinical trial
- Observation
- Same treatment as before or different treatment from before

When cancer appears resistant to multiple therapies, it is called refractory. For refractory disease, a clinical trial or brentuximab vedotin are options.

Guide 9 Primary treatment options: Widespread lesions
Observation (preferred if asymptomatic)
Methotrexate
Phototherapy
Systemic retinoids
Topical steroids
Topical mechlorethamine (nitrogen mustard)

No response

If no response or refractory disease, then the options are:

> Clinical trial

> Another treatment not used before

For refractory disease, the options are:

> Clinical trial

> Brentuximab vedotin

Monitoring

Those with LyP are at risk for developing another type of lymphoma. Life-long follow-up will be needed. Your doctor should conduct a thorough skin exam during each follow-up visit. Ask how you will be monitored and how often you should have a check-up.

Review

> Lymphomatoid papulosis (LyP) is a benign, chronic, recurring disease of the immune system.

> LyP is not cancer. Treatment includes skin-directed and/or systemic therapy. A clinical trial may be an option.

> Observation is preferred for those without symptoms (asymptomatic).

> Treatment for widespread or extensive lesions aims to reduce the number of lesions and any discomfort they may cause.

> When cancer appears resistant to multiple therapies, it is called refractory.

> Those with LyP are at risk for developing another type of lymphoma. Ongoing monitoring will be needed.

8
Making treatment decisions

57   It's your choice

58   Questions to ask your doctors

67   Resources

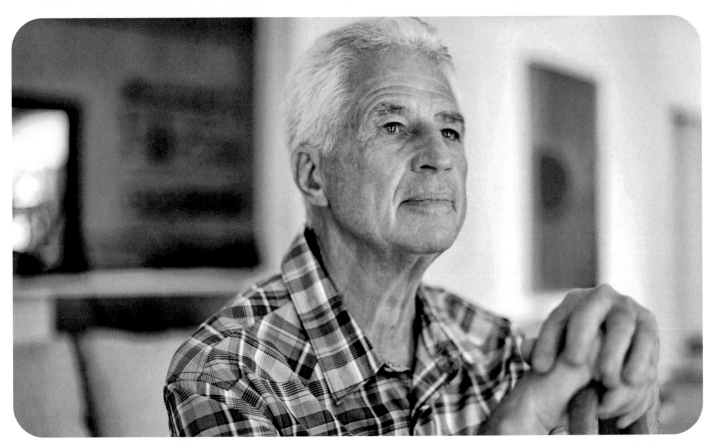

It's important to be comfortable with the cancer treatment you choose. This choice starts with having an open and honest conversation with your doctor.

It's your choice

In shared decision-making, you and your doctors share information, discuss the options, and agree on a treatment plan. It starts with an open and honest conversation between you and your doctor.

Treatment decisions are very personal. What is important to you may not be important to someone else.

Some things that may play a role in your decision-making:

> What you want and how that might differ from what others want

> Your religious and spiritual beliefs

> Your feelings about certain treatments like surgery or chemotherapy

> Your feelings about pain or side effects such as nausea and vomiting

> Cost of treatment, travel to treatment centers, and time away from school or work

> Quality of life and length of life

> How active you are and the activities that are important to you

Think about what you want from treatment. Discuss openly the risks and benefits of specific treatments and procedures. Weigh options and share concerns with your doctor. If you take the

time to build a relationship with your doctor, it will help you feel supported when considering options and making treatment decisions.

Second opinion

It is normal to want to start treatment as soon as possible. While cancer can't be ignored, there is time to have another doctor review your test results and suggest a treatment plan. This is called getting a second opinion, and it's a normal part of cancer care. Even doctors get second opinions!

Things you can do to prepare:

> Check with your insurance company about its rules on second opinions. There may be out-of-pocket costs to see doctors who are not part of your insurance plan.

> Make plans to have copies of all your records sent to the doctor you will see for your second opinion.

Support groups

Many people diagnosed with cancer find support groups to be helpful. Support groups often include people at different stages of treatment. Some people may be newly diagnosed, while others may be finished with treatment. If your hospital or community doesn't have support groups for people with cancer, check out the websites listed in this book.

Questions to ask your doctors

Possible questions to ask your doctors are listed on the following pages. Feel free to use these questions or come up with your own. Be clear about your goals for treatment and find out what to expect from treatment.

Questions to ask about testing and staging

1. What type of cancer do I have? What is the cancer stage? What does this mean?

2. Is it in my blood? Lymph nodes? Other organs?

3. When will I have a biopsy? What type of biopsy? What are the risks?

4. Is there a cancer center or hospital nearby that specializes in this type of cancer?

5. What tests are needed? What other tests do you recommend? Will I have any genetic or molecular tests?

6. What will you do to make me comfortable during testing?

7. How do I prepare for testing? How and where will the test be done?

8. How soon will I know the results and who will explain them to me?

9. Would you give me a copy of the pathology report and other test results?

10. Who will talk with me about the next steps? When?

11. Will treatment start before the test results are in?

12. Can my cancer be cured? If not, how well can treatment stop the cancer from growing?

Questions to ask about skin

1. Is this cancer contagious? Will it spread to people who touch me?

2. Should I avoid sharing clothes or towels? How often should I change or wash towels?

3. Can I use lotions or oils on my skin or hair other than what you give me? What about the best types of soap or shampoo? Hair dye? Makeup?

4. Is it better to wear long sleeves, pants, or cover the rash/lesions in some way? Or should I let them be exposed to the air as much as possible?

5. Should I take time to inspect my skin? If so, how often?

6. If I notice any changes in my skin whom should I call? When?

7. Will keeping a diary and photo journal help? What should I include in the diary? How often should I take photos?

8. Can I go out in the sun? Should I wear sunscreen? Long sleeves? Hat?

9. Are there any changes that I can make to my diet? Exercise?

10. What about stress? Will stress worsen my condition?

Questions to ask your doctors about their experience

1. What is your experience treating this type of cancer?

2. What is the experience of those on your team?

3. What types of cancer do you treat?

4. I would like to get a second opinion. Is there someone you recommend?

5. How many patients like me (of the same age, gender, race) have you treated?

6. Will you be consulting with experts to discuss my care? Whom will you consult?

7. How many procedures like the one you're suggesting have you done?

8. Is this treatment a major part of your practice?

9. How many of your patients have had complications? What were the complications?

10. Who will manage my day-to-day care?

Questions to ask about treatment

1. Which treatment do you recommend and why? Is this treatment a cure? What are the benefits and risks?

2. How long do I have to decide?

3. Will I have to go to the hospital or elsewhere for treatment? How often? How long is each visit? Will I have to stay overnight in the hospital or make travel plans?

4. Do I have a choice of when to begin treatment? Can I choose the days and times of treatment?

5. How much will the treatment hurt? What will you do to make me comfortable?

6. How much will this treatment cost? What does my insurance cover? Are there any programs to help pay for treatment?

7. What kind of treatment will I do at home? What can I do to prepare my home to ensure my safety or the safety of other family members in the household? What type of home care will I need?

8. Are there any life-threatening side effects of this treatment? How will these be monitored?

9. What should I expect from this treatment? How long will treatment last?

10. How do you know if treatment is working? How will I know if treatment is working?

11. What in particular should be avoided or taken with caution while receiving treatment?

12. What are the chances my cancer will return? Am I at risk for developing another kind of cancer, such as skin cancer?

Questions to ask about biopsies

1. What kind of biopsy will I have? Will I have more than one biopsy?

2. What types of tests will be done on the biopsy sample? What will you look for?

3. What will be removed during the biopsy?

4. How long will it take me to recover?

5. How much pain will I be in? What will be done to manage my pain?

6. What other side effects can I expect?

Questions to ask about radiation therapy

1. What type of radiation therapy (RT) will I have? How is this different from other types of RT?

2. What are the risks of this treatment?

3. What will you target?

4. What is the goal of this radiation treatment? Will RT be used with other therapies?

5. How many treatment sessions will I require? Can you do a shorter course of radiation?

6. Will I need someone to drive me home after treatment? What can I expect from treatment?

7. Do you offer this type of radiation here? If not, can you refer me to someone who does?

8. What side effects can I expect from radiation? How will these be treated?

Questions to ask about clinical trials

1. What clinical trials are available? Am I eligible for any of them? Why or why not?

2. What are the treatments used in the clinical trial?

3. What does the treatment do?

4. Has the treatment been used before? Has it been used for other types of cancer?

5. What are the risks and benefits of this treatment?

6. What side effects should I expect? How will the side effects be controlled?

7. How long will I be on the clinical trial?

8. Will I be able to get other treatment if this doesn't work?

9. How will you know the treatment is working?

10. Will the clinical trial cost me anything? If so, how much?

Questions to ask about side effects

1. What are the side effects of treatment?

2. How long will these side effects last? Do any side effects lessen or worsen in severity over time?

3. What side effects should I watch for? What side effects are expected and which are life threatening?

4. When should I call the doctor? Can I text?

5. What medicines can I take to prevent or relieve side effects?

6. What can I do to help with pain and other side effects?

7. Will you stop treatment or change treatment if there are side effects? What do you look for?

8. What can I do to lessen or prevent side effects? What will you do?

9. What side effects are life-long and irreversible even after completing treatment?

10. What medicines may worsen side effects of treatment?

Questions to ask about survivorship and late effects

1. What happens after treatment?

2. What are the chances cancer will return or I will get another type of cancer?

3. Who do I see for follow-up care? How often? For how many years?

4. What should I do if I have trouble paying for follow-up visits and tests?

5. What tests will I have to monitor my health?

6. What late effects are caused by this treatment? How will these be screened?

7. I am looking for a survivor support group. What support groups or other resources can you recommend?

8. What happens if I move after treatment and have to change doctors? Will you help me find a doctor?

Resources

American Academy of Dermatology Association (AADA)
aad.org/public

American Cancer Society (ACS)
Cancer.org

Cancer Hope Network
Cancerhopenetwork.org

Cutaneous Lymphoma Foundation (CLF)
clfoundation.org

International Society for Cutaneous Lymphomas (ISCL)
cutaneouslymphoma.org

Leukemia & Lymphoma Society (LLS)
LLS.org/informationspecialists

Lymphoma Research Foundation
lymphoma.org/aboutlymphoma/nhl/cbcl

lymphoma.org/aboutlymphoma/nhl/ctcl

National Cancer Institute (NCI)
cancer.gov/types/lymphoma/patient/mycosis-fungoides-treatment-pdq

How monoclonal antibodies treat cancer

National Coalition for Cancer Survivorship
canceradvocacy.org/toolbox

National Organization for Rare Diseases (NORD)
rarediseases.org

The Skin of Color Society (SOCS)
skinofcolorsociety.org

VisualDx
skinsight.com askaysa.com

Words to know

biopsy
The removal of a sample of tissue for testing.

blood tumor burden
The amount of cancerous cells in the blood.

chemotherapy
Drugs that kill fast-growing cells, including cancer cells and normal cells.

clinical trial
A type of research that assesses health tests or treatments.

complete blood count (CBC)
A lab test that includes the number of blood cells.

dermatologist
A doctor who specializes in the diagnosis and treatment of skin diseases.

external beam radiation therapy (EBRT)
A cancer treatment with radiation received from a machine outside the body.

gene
Coded instructions in cells for making new cells and controlling how cells behave.

histology
The structure of cells, tissue, and organs as viewed under a microscope.

imaging test
A test that makes pictures (images) of the insides of the body.

immune system
The body's natural defense against infection and disease.

immunohistochemistry (IHC)
A lab test of cancer cells to find specific cell traits involved in abnormal cell growth.

involved-site radiation therapy (ISRT)
Targets a specific area of skin. It can also be used to treat specific lymph nodes with cancer.

lymph
A clear fluid containing white blood cells.

lymphadenopathy
Lymph nodes that are abnormal in size or consistency.

lymphatic system
Germ-fighting network of tissues and organs that includes the bone marrow, spleen, thymus, lymph nodes, and lymphatic vessels. Part of the immune system.

lymph node
A small, bean-shaped, disease-fighting structure.

medical oncologist
A doctor who is an expert in cancer drugs.

pallor
Skin that is paler than usual.

palpable adenopathy
Lymph nodes that feel abnormal in size or consistency.

papule
A small, solid, raised bump on the skin that might look like small pimples. Papules may be red, purple, brown, or pink.

papulonodular
Combination of papules and nodules found on the skin.

patch
A flat, thin, pink or red skin lesion of any size.

pathologist
A doctor who is an expert in testing cells and tissue to find disease.

persistent
Cancer that remains or returns.

phototherapy
uses different ultraviolet (UV) light wavelengths to treat skin lesions or tumors.

plaque
A raised (elevated) or hardened (indurated) skin lesion of any size.

progression
The growth or spread of cancer after being tested or treated.

radiation oncologist
A doctor who's an expert in treating cancer with radiation.

radiation therapy (RT)
A treatment that uses high-energy rays or related approaches to kill cancer cells.

refractory
Cancer that does not respond to multiple treatments.

regression
A decrease in the size of a patch, plaque, or tumor or the amount of cancer in the body.

relapse
The return or worsening of cancer after a period of improvement.

remission
There are minor or no signs of disease.

retinoids
Products related to vitamin A.

scale
When the outer layer of skin peels away in large pieces.

side effect
An unhealthy or unpleasant physical or emotional response to treatment.

skin-directed therapy
Treatment focused on the skin. Includes topical therapy, local radiation, and phototherapy.

skin disease burden
The amount of cancerous cells found in the skin.

supportive care
Health care that includes symptom relief but not cancer treatment. Also called palliative care or best supportive care.

systemic therapy
Treatment that works throughout the body.

targeted therapy
A drug treatment that targets and attacks specific cancer cells.

total skin electron beam therapy (TSEBT)
Treats the entire skin surface.

NCCN Contributors

This patient guide is based on the NCCN Clinical Practice Guidelines in Oncology (NCCN Guidelines®) for Primary Cutaneous Lymphomas, Version 1.2021. It was adapted, reviewed, and published with help from the following people:

Dorothy A. Shead, MS
Director, Patient Information Operations

Rachael Clarke
Senior Medical Copyeditor

Tanya Fischer, MEd, MSLIS
Medical Writer

Laura J. Hanisch, PsyD
Medical Writer/Patient Information Specialist

Stephanie Helbling, MPH, CHES®
Medical Writer

Susan Kidney
Graphic Design Specialist

John Murphy
Medical Writer

Erin Vidic, MA
Medical Writer

Kim Williams
Creative Services Manager

The NCCN Guidelines® for Primary Cutaneous Lymphomas, Version 1.2021, were developed by the following NCCN Panel Members:

***Steven M. Horwitz, MD/Chair**
Memorial Sloan Kettering Cancer Center

***Stephen Ansell, MD, PhD/Vice-Chair**
Mayo Clinic Cancer Center

Weiyun Z. Ai, MD, PhD
UCSF Helen Diller Family Comprehensive Cancer Center

Jeffrey Barnes, MD, PhD
Massachusetts General Hospital Cancer Center

Stefan K. Barta, MD, MRCP, MS
Abramson Cancer Center at the University of Pennsylvania

Mark W. Clemens, MD
The University of Texas MD Anderson Cancer Center

Ahmet Dogan, MD, PhD
Memorial Sloan Kettering Cancer Center

Aaron M. Goodman, MD
UC San Diego Moores Cancer Center

Gaurav Goyal, MD
O'Neal Comprehensive Cancer Center at UAB

***Joan Guitart, MD**
Robert H. Lurie Comprehensive Cancer Center of Northwestern University

Ahmad Halwani, MD
Huntsman Cancer Institute at the University of Utah

***Bradley M. Haverkos, MD, MPH, MS**
University of Colorado Cancer Center

***Richard T. Hoppe, MD**
Stanford Cancer Institute

Eric Jacobsen, MD
Dana-Farber/Brigham and Women's Cancer Center

Deepa Jagadeesh, MD, MPH
Case Comprehensive Cancer Center/ University Hospitals Seidman Cancer Center and Cleveland Clinic Taussig Cancer Institute

Allison Jones
St. Jude Children's Research Hospital/ The University of Tennessee Health Science Center

Youn H. Kim, MD
Stanford Cancer Institute

Neha Mehta-Shah, MD
Siteman Cancer Center at Barnes-Jewish Hospital and Washington University School of Medicine

Elise A. Olsen, MD
Duke Cancer Institute

Barbara Pro, MD
Robert H. Lurie Comprehensive Cancer Center of Northwestern University

Saurabh A. Rajguru, MD
University of Wisconsin Carbone Cancer Center

Sima Rozati, MD, PhD
The Sidney Kimmel Comprehensive Cancer Center at Johns Hopkins

***Jonathan Said, MD**
UCLA Jonsson Comprehensive Cancer Center

Aaron Shaver, MD, PhD
Vanderbilt-Ingram Cancer Center

Andrei Shustov, MD
Fred Hutchinson Cancer Research Center/ Seattle Cancer Care Alliance

Lubomir Sokol, MD, PhD
Moffitt Cancer Center

Pallawi Torka, MD
Roswell Park Cancer Institute

Carlos Torres-Cabala, MD
The University of Texas MD Anderson Cancer Center

Ryan Wilcox, MD, PhD
University of Michigan Rogel Cancer Center

Basem M. William, MD
The Ohio State University Comprehensive Cancer Center - James Cancer Hospital and Solove Research Institute

Jasmine Zain, MD
City of Hope National Medical Center

NCCN

Mary Dwyer, MS
Director, Guidelines Operations

Hema Sundar, PhD
Manager, Global Clinical Content

* Reviewed this patient guide. For disclosures, visit NCCN.org/about/disclosure.aspx.

NCCN Cancer Centers

Abramson Cancer Center
at the University of Pennsylvania
Philadelphia, Pennsylvania
800.789.7366 • pennmedicine.org/cancer

Fred & Pamela Buffett Cancer Center
Omaha, Nebraska
402.559.5600 • unmc.edu/cancercenter

Case Comprehensive Cancer Center/
University Hospitals Seidman Cancer
Center and Cleveland Clinic Taussig
Cancer Institute
Cleveland, Ohio
800.641.2422 • UH Seidman Cancer Center
uhhospitals.org/services/cancer-services
866.223.8100 • CC Taussig Cancer Institute
my.clevelandclinic.org/departments/cancer
216.844.8797 • Case CCC
case.edu/cancer

City of Hope National Medical Center
Los Angeles, California
800.826.4673 • cityofhope.org

Dana-Farber/Brigham and
Women's Cancer Center |
Massachusetts General Hospital
Cancer Center
Boston, Massachusetts
617.732.5500
youhaveus.org
617.726.5130
massgeneral.org/cancer-center

Duke Cancer Institute
Durham, North Carolina
888.275.3853 • dukecancerinstitute.org

Fox Chase Cancer Center
Philadelphia, Pennsylvania
888.369.2427 • foxchase.org

Huntsman Cancer Institute
at the University of Utah
Salt Lake City, Utah
800.824.2073
huntsmancancer.org

Fred Hutchinson Cancer
Research Center/Seattle
Cancer Care Alliance
Seattle, Washington
206.606.7222 • seattlecca.org
206.667.5000 • fredhutch.org

The Sidney Kimmel Comprehensive
Cancer Center at Johns Hopkins
Baltimore, Maryland
410.955.8964
www.hopkinskimmelcancercenter.org

Robert H. Lurie Comprehensive
Cancer Center of Northwestern
University
Chicago, Illinois
866.587.4322 • cancer.northwestern.edu

Mayo Clinic Cancer Center
Phoenix/Scottsdale, Arizona
Jacksonville, Florida
Rochester, Minnesota
480.301.8000 • Arizona
904.953.0853 • Florida
507.538.3270 • Minnesota
mayoclinic.org/cancercenter

Memorial Sloan Kettering
Cancer Center
New York, New York
800.525.2225 • mskcc.org

Moffitt Cancer Center
Tampa, Florida
888.663.3488 • moffitt.org

The Ohio State University
Comprehensive Cancer Center -
James Cancer Hospital and
Solove Research Institute
Columbus, Ohio
800.293.5066 • cancer.osu.edu

O'Neal Comprehensive
Cancer Center at UAB
Birmingham, Alabama
800.822.0933 • uab.edu/onealcancercenter

Roswell Park Comprehensive
Cancer Center
Buffalo, New York
877.275.7724 • roswellpark.org

Siteman Cancer Center at Barnes-
Jewish Hospital and Washington
University School of Medicine
St. Louis, Missouri
800.600.3606 • siteman.wustl.edu

St. Jude Children's Research Hospital/
The University of Tennessee
Health Science Center
Memphis, Tennessee
866.278.5833 • stjude.org
901.448.5500 • uthsc.edu

Stanford Cancer Institute
Stanford, California
877.668.7535 • cancer.stanford.edu

UC San Diego Moores Cancer Center
La Jolla, California
858.822.6100• cancer.ucsd.edu

UCLA Jonsson
Comprehensive Cancer Center
Los Angeles, California
310.825.5268 • cancer.ucla.edu

UCSF Helen Diller Family
Comprehensive Cancer Center
San Francisco, California
800.689.8273 • cancer.ucsf.edu

University of Colorado Cancer Center
Aurora, Colorado
720.848.0300 • coloradocancercenter.org

University of Michigan
Rogel Cancer Center
Ann Arbor, Michigan
800.865.1125 • rogelcancercenter.org

The University of Texas
MD Anderson Cancer Center
Houston, Texas
844.269.5922 • mdanderson.org

University of Wisconsin
Carbone Cancer Center
Madison, Wisconsin
608.265.1700 • uwhealth.org/cancer

UT Southwestern Simmons
Comprehensive Cancer Center
Dallas, Texas
214.648.3111 • utsouthwestern.edu/simmons

Vanderbilt-Ingram Cancer Center
Nashville, Tennessee
877.936.8422 • vicc.org

Yale Cancer Center/
Smilow Cancer Hospital
New Haven, Connecticut
855.4.SMILOW • yalecancercenter.org

Notes

ALK 20–21

anaplastic large cell lymphoma (ALCL) 10, 42–50

B cell (or B lymphocyte) 8–9

biomarkers 21–22

biopsy 1–19

CD30-positive (CD30+) 42–46

chemotherapy 28

clinical trials 30

cutaneous ALCL 45–50

cutaneous B-cell lymphoma (CBCL) 9, 33–40

cutaneous T-cell lymphoma (CTCL) 10, 43

external beam radiation therapy (EBRT) 28

gene rearrangements 21

immunotherapy 28

involved-site radiation therapy (ISRT) 28

local therapy 27

lymph node 7–8, 19, 23

lymphocytes 8

lymphomatoid papulosis (LyP) 53–55

lymphoproliferative disorder (LPD) 10, 42

molecular testing 21–22

phototherapy 28

primary cutaneous anaplastic large cell lymphoma (PC-ALCL) 47–48

primary cutaneous CD30+ T-cell lymphoproliferative disorder (PCLPD) 42–46

primary cutaneous lymphoma (PCL) 9

primary cutaneous diffuse large B-cell lymphoma (PC-DLBCL), leg type 9, 34–35

primary cutaneous follicle center lymphoma (PCFCL) 9, 34–40

primary cutaneous marginal zone lymphoma (PCMZL) 9, 34–40

radiation therapy (RT) 28

retinoids 28

skin-directed therapy 27

skin exam 15

T cell (or T lymphocyte) 8–10

targeted therapy 28

TCR 21, 43

topical therapy 27

total skin electron beam therapy (TSEBT) 28

Made in the USA
Middletown, DE
16 September 2021